ALMOST
ADDICTED

ALMOST ADDICTED

Is My (or My Loved One's) Drug Use a Problem?

J. Wesley Boyd, MD, PhD, Harvard Medical School

with Eric Metcalf, MPH

HAZELDEN®

Hazelden
Center City, Minnesota 55012
hazelden.org

Library of Congress Cataloging-in-Publication Data

Boyd, J. Wesley (Jon Wesley)
    Almost addicted : is my (or my loved one's) drug use a problem? /
J. Wesley Boyd with Eric Metcalf.
        p. cm.
    Includes bibliographical references.
    ISBN 978-1-61649-101-7 (softcover)
    1. Drug abuse—Psychological aspects. 2. Drug abuse—Prevention.
3. Substance abuse—Psychological aspects. 4. Substance abuse—
Prevention. 5. Addicts—Rehabilitation. I. Metcalf, Eric. II. Title.
    RC564.B69 2012
    616.86—dc23

                                                    2012023939

Editor's notes:
The case examples in this book are composite examples based upon
behaviors encountered in the author's own professional experience. None
of the individuals described in this book are based on a specific patient,
and all identifying details in the composite examples have been changed
to protect the privacy of the people involved.

    This publication is not intended as a substitute for the advice of
health care professionals.

    Alcoholics Anonymous and AA are registered trademarks of Alcoholics
Anonymous World Services, Inc.

16 15 14 13 12   1 2 3 4 5 6

Cover design by Theresa Jaeger Gedig
Interior design and typesetting by Kinne Design

Harvard Health Publications
HARVARD MEDICAL SCHOOL
Trusted advice for a healthier life

The Almost Effect™ **series** presents books written
by Harvard Medical School faculty and other
experts who offer guidance on common behavioral
and physical problems falling in the spectrum between
normal health and a full-blown medical condition.
These are the first publications to help general readers
recognize and address these problems.

Wesley Boyd dedicates this book to his wife, Theonia, and to his children, Naomi, Ariana, Anaïs, and Emerson.

Eric Metcalf dedicates this book to his wife, Brie, and houseful of kids, Milo, Rak, and Ellie.

contents

The Almost Effect

I once overheard a mother counseling her grown daughter to avoid dating a man she thought had a drinking problem. The daughter said, "Mom, he's not an alcoholic!" The mother quickly responded, "Well, maybe not, but he *almost* is."

Perhaps you've heard someone, referring to a boss or public figure, say, "I don't like that guy. He's *almost* a psychopath!"

Over the years, I've heard many variations on this theme. The medical literature currently recognizes many problems or syndromes that don't quite meet the standard definition of a medical condition. Although the medical literature has many examples of these syndromes, they are often not well known (except by doctors specializing in that particular area of medicine) or well described (except in highly technical medical research articles). They are what medical professionals often refer to as subclinical and, using the common parlance from the examples above, what we're calling *the almost effect*.

For example:

- Glucose intolerance may not always lead to the medical condition of diabetes, but it nonetheless increases your risk of getting diabetes—which then increases your risk of heart attacks, strokes, and many other illnesses.

- Sunburns, especially severe ones, may not always lead to skin cancer, but they always increase your risk of skin cancer, cause immediate pain, and may cause permanent cosmetic issues.

- Pre-hypertension may not always lead to hypertension (high blood pressure), but it increases your risk of getting hypertension, which then increases your risk of heart attacks, strokes, and other illnesses.

- Osteopenia signifies a minor loss of bone that may not always lead to the more significant bone loss called osteoporosis, but it still increases your risk of getting osteoporosis, which then increases your risk of having a pathologic fracture.

Diseases can develop slowly, producing milder symptoms for years before they become full-blown. If you recognize them early, before they become fully developed, and take relatively simple actions, you have a good chance of preventing them from turning into the full-blown disorder. In many instances there are steps you can try at home on your own; this is especially true with the mental and behavioral health disorders.

So, what exactly is the almost effect and why this book? *Almost Addicted* is one of a series of books by faculty members from Harvard Medical School and other experts. These books are the first to describe in everyday language how to recognize and what to do about some of the most common behavioral and emotional problems that fall within the continuum between normal and full-blown pathology. Since this concept is new and still evolving, we're proposing a new term, *the almost effect*, to describe problems characterized by the following criteria.

The problem

1. falls outside of normal behavior but falls short of meeting the criteria for a particular diagnosis (such as alcoholism, major depression, psychopathy, or substance dependence);

2. is currently causing identifiable issues for individuals and/or others in their lives;

3. may progress to the full-blown condition, meeting accepted diagnostic criteria, but even if it doesn't, still can cause significant suffering;

4. should respond to appropriate interventions when accurately identified.

The Almost Effect

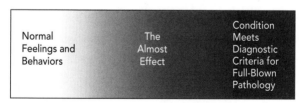

| Normal Feelings and Behaviors | The Almost Effect | Condition Meets Diagnostic Criteria for Full-Blown Pathology |

All of the books in The Almost Effect™ series make a simple point: Each of these conditions occurs along a spectrum, with normal health and behavior at one end and the full-blown disorder at the other. Between these two extremes is where the almost effect lies. It is the point at which a person is experiencing real pain and suffering from a condition for which there are solutions—*if* the problem is recognized.

Recognizing the almost effect not only helps a person address real issues now, it also opens the door for change well in advance of the point at which the problem becomes severe. In short, recognizing the almost effect has two primary goals: (1) to alleviate pain and suffering now and (2) to prevent more serious problems later.

I am convinced these problems are causing tremendous suffering, and it is my hope that the science-based information in these books can help alleviate this suffering. Readers can find help in the practical self-assessments and advice offered here, and the current research and clinical expertise presented in the series can open opportunities for health care professionals to intervene more effectively.

I hope you find this book helpful. For information about other books in this series, visit www.TheAlmostEffect.com.

Julie Silver, MD
Assistant Professor, Harvard Medical School
Chief Editor of Books, Harvard Health Publications

acknowledgments

Wesley Boyd would like to thank the many people who have made this book possible. First, he thanks his many amazing teachers over the years who taught him much and also held the bar very high: Jeffry Andresen, Larry Churchill, Bill Peck, Leston Havens, John Mack, Myron Sharaf, Bennett Simon, and Hal Borus. He has also learned a tremendous amount from the patients he has worked with, as well as from the many students and residents he has known.

He also owes much gratitude to Sid Farrar, Natalie Ramm, Linda Konner, and especially Julie Silver, without whom this book simply wouldn't have happened. He was also blessed to be introduced to Eric Metcalf, whose talents, knowledge, and experience have made this book far better than it would have otherwise been.

His mother, Frida Boyd, has helped tremendously with household and child care duties over many years, which in turn has allowed him to throw himself into professional endeavors much more so than he might have.

And finally, he owes more than he can convey to his wife, Theonia Boyd, who is his running partner as well as his partner in life, confidante, and unerring bearer of sage advice.

. . .

Eric Metcalf would like to thank his wife, Brie, for her patience, encouragement, and good humor, and his parents, Earl and Marcia, and the rest of his family for their unflagging support. He's also grateful to the many people who developed and guided this project. Special thanks to Wesley Boyd for the insight and spirit of collaboration he brought to this book.

■◆■

| introduction |

Almost Addicted: The Basics

In my years as a psychiatrist, nearly all of the people I have encountered who used marijuana swore to me that their pot smoking wasn't harmful. That's because, as far as they could tell, it never caused any problems in their work, school performance, health, or well-being. To the contrary, they were convinced that their lives were actually *better* because of marijuana use, even if those around them told them otherwise.

People who use marijuana often relieve any guilt about smoking it by adopting the philosophy that, because marijuana is a natural substance, it's not a drug. Just for good measure, they will often throw in the fact that marijuana has been legalized or decriminalized in some states. As a result, many people who use marijuana have no intention of cutting back.

But people who smoke pot aren't alone. Drinkers who look forward to several beers at night to relax or people who snort a few lines of coke at a party several times a year so they can be part of the action have their own lines of defense.

These folks often reassure themselves that they don't have a problem with their substance use because they, like everybody else, know what someone with a "true addiction" looks like and their use doesn't compare. When they picture a person with a *true* addiction, they're probably picturing someone whose life is visibly unstable—like these examples of addiction I have encountered over the years:

- The marijuana smoker who maintained his construction job but who smoked all day every day, lacked the motivation to do anything other than show up for work, and readily told me, "Marijuana is my hobby, my girlfriend, my retirement account—pretty much *everything* except work."

- The man who takes 200 milligrams (mg) of OxyContin daily and whose life revolves around ensuring that he always has a steady supply of the drug. More than anything in the world, he lives in dread of his system running out of the drug, leaving him in withdrawal. Because OxyContin is costly on the street, this person has committed numerous crimes over the years to support his habit, including selling his family's heirloom jewelry and stealing cash from his grandmother, who lives off her Social Security payments.

- The alcoholic who clutches a vodka bottle in his fist day and night and sips from it liberally as he wanders the streets. He stumbles and slurs his words, reeking of alcohol. Repeatedly refusing his friends' offers to come in off the streets, he chooses instead to sleep under an overpass with all the other "bums" like him.

- The beautiful young woman who has been using heroin every day for a year with a group of her "friends" and has been repeatedly sexually assaulted while passed out after getting high.

- A drug-addicted physician who always shows up for work, takes (reasonably) good care of her patients, and keeps her drug of choice in her office desk drawer, using it throughout the work day to ensure that she doesn't go into withdrawal.

Each person is undeniably drug dependent, and in almost twenty years of psychiatric practice, I have seen many other individuals with stories like these. I've worked with people from all walks of life—whether poor, working class, or well-to-do—and I've treated patients with a full range of addictive behaviors in each of these groups.

After medical school, I trained as a resident in psychiatry at the Cambridge Hospital, a public hospital in Massachusetts affiliated with Harvard Medical School. Since then, I have worked in a multitude of other settings, including private practice, public and private hospitals, addiction clinics for adults, an addiction clinic for teenagers, academic and community facilities, and even a program that assists doctors with substance use disorders. Through it all, I've worked with more patients while on night and weekend shifts than I can remember.

For the past eight years, I have been back at Cambridge Health Alliance (the expanded network that includes Cambridge Hospital), where I work as part of a general adult psychiatric teaching team that specializes in patients who have substance use disorders in addition to general psychiatric issues. I am also a staff psychiatrist at Children's Hospital Boston in its adolescent substance abuse program.

Across these various settings, in addition to the people with true addiction depicted above, I have also seen many individuals whose occasional drug use didn't appear to be a problem. These are the people who now and then can use drugs, whether legal or illicit, yet not experience any trouble as a result.

But between these people who can take drugs occasionally without incident and those with hard-core addiction is another important group: the "almost addicted." These are the individuals whose drug use does not rise to the level that would meet the criteria for a formal diagnosis of addiction but who nonetheless are suffering to some extent from their drug-related behaviors.

Drug use among the almost addicted falls outside of normal behavior but doesn't quite meet any diagnostic criteria for drug abuse. Still, this type of drug use causes real problems in the moment for either these individuals or those around them. If left unchecked, it might progress to full-blown addiction. For these reasons, identifying almost addiction and taking measures to change the behavior is vital. This is why I am writing this book.

Think about it: even if you don't have a full-blown addiction and you haven't had major difficulties in your life because of substance abuse, your drug use can still negatively impact your life. You can still have a "drug problem." Indeed, I believe that there is a huge swath of people out there who are almost addicted.

If you have an image of what a person with a true addiction looks like, how do you identify someone with an *almost* addiction?

It's not always easy. A stranger would never readily identify someone who is almost addicted as a person with a drug problem. When people chat about America's problems with drugs, the image of those who are almost addicted isn't what comes to their minds. It isn't hard to understand why some people (including many health care professionals) conclude that there are only two kinds of people in the world: addicts and nonaddicts. If you were to draw a picture of such a vision of "the drug-using world," it would look like this:

The Drug-Using World

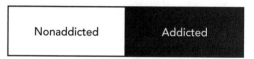

Yet in reality the drug-using world is not so black and white. Being *addicted* to, or *dependent* on, a substance is different from *abusing* a substance (we'll discuss that difference a bit later). Although many people use drugs to obtain a buzz, relax, or otherwise feel good, people who are *almost* addicted go beyond occasional use and cross into a gray area—the territory in which problems arise because of drug use. Examples include the following:

- People who only feel good when they are under the influence and who get irritable when they don't have a drug in their system
- Those who occasionally fail to show up for functions and obligations because they're high
- People whose school or work performance has fallen off because of drug use

- Anyone who is experiencing a lack of intimacy or conflicts in relationships with family members, friends, spouses, or co-workers that can be tied to increased drug use

Indeed, experts have come to view the world of drug users as not sharply divided into two types of people, but rather as consisting of a wide diversity of people. Thus, the drug-using world looks something like this:

The Drug-Using World

| Nonaddicted (Nonusers and occasional users) | Almost Addicted | Addicted |

The Numbers

Just how many people are almost addicted? According to the most recent and probably best estimate of illicit drug use, 21.8 million Americans age twelve or older (or 8.7 percent) had used illicit drugs in the month before the 2009 survey. This group had grown by 9 percent from the previous year.[1]

In 2009, 16.7 million people ages twelve and older in the United States had used marijuana at least once in the previous month.[2] Kids and teens account for many of the users among that "twelve and older" group. A 2010 large-scale study from the University of Michigan found that 13.7 percent of eighth graders, 27.5 percent of tenth graders, and 34.8 percent of twelfth graders had used marijuana at least once in the year before being surveyed.[3]

In terms of prescription drug abuse—which involves substances such as pain relievers, tranquilizers, stimulants, or sedatives—in 2009, 16 million people in the United States used these drugs for nonmedical purposes at least once in the past year.[4] As with marijuana, when it comes to opiate pain-killers, youth are certainly getting in on the act. The University of Michigan study cited earlier also found that 2.7 percent of eighth graders and 8 percent of twelfth graders had abused Vicodin, and 2.1 percent of eighth graders and 5.1 percent of twelfth graders had abused OxyContin within the previous year.[5]

By no means is the United States alone in its appetite for street drugs and the nonmedical use of prescription drugs. For example, recent reports found that in 2009–2010 in England and Wales, 8.6 percent of adults had used illicit drugs in the previous year. In England, 22 percent of eleven- to fifteen-year-olds had used a drug at least once in their lives. For both groups, marijuana was the most widely used drug.[6] In Germany, a 2006 survey found that 5.4 percent of adults had used illegal drugs in the previous year, and nearly one-quarter had used illegal drugs at least once in their lives (again, the drug of choice was most often marijuana).[7]

So many millions of people, young and old, are using illegal drugs worldwide. Do most of them fit the stereotypical image of the dysfunctional, hustling "addict" who can't fit into normal society? Of course not. Most are occasional users who have few if any negative effects. But what about people who use drugs regularly? Although a small portion of these individuals are undoubtedly dependent on drugs, and a slightly larger number would fall into the substance abuse category, the vast majority of these folks fit the definition of what you could call almost addicted.

This book is intended to help the vast number of people who are not substance dependent but who nonetheless show what doctors call "maladaptive use," which is drug use that causes harm.

Types of Drugs

When people talk about *drugs*, what exactly are they referring to? Although intoxicants might be classified in many different ways, in general there are three broad categories: stimulants, depressants, and hallucinogens. Each type of drug brings with it different perceived rewards for users, as well as different downsides. The legality of the drugs I'm discussing in this book varies: some may be illegal in any setting, such as heroin; others may be legal in some situations, as is the case with prescription medications, but are being used for purposes or in amounts other than the doctor intended; and still others may exist in a legally gray area in some locations, such as marijuana.

Stimulants

Stimulants are drugs that generally speed people up and make them feel happy or even elated. They can also increase heart rate and blood pressure, as well as cause anxiety and panic. This category of drugs includes cocaine in its various forms (powder or crack). Cocaine is virtually never used for medical purposes and is essentially illegal everywhere drugs are prohibited.

Other drugs in this category include amphetamine-based preparations, among them drugs such as Adderall, Vyvanse, and Dexedrine. Another category of stimulants includes the methylphenidate-based drugs: Ritalin, Concerta, Focalin,

Metadate, and other specific drugs. Amphetamine- and methyl-phenidate-based drugs are produced in various forms, including short-acting, long-acting, or even combination pills. While these drugs are legitimately used to treat attention-deficit hyperactivity disorder, they are also abused because they can cause mood changes and feelings of elation. Some people who abuse them crush the drugs and snort them to get a more rapid rush of euphoric feelings.

Crystal meth, short for methamphetamine, is a highly potent and highly addictive form of amphetamine. Similar to the impact of crack cocaine, crystal meth has devastated individuals, families, and communities because of its powerfully addictive properties and the damage it leaves in its path.

Even though people use stimulants for the euphoric high that they trigger, as the drugs wear off, users can feel extremely lethargic and depressed and lack the motivation to do much of anything.

Depressants

Depressant drugs are used by individuals who want to feel calmer, zone out for a while, or relax. Not surprisingly, the substances in this category slow many bodily processes, such as heart rate. They also decrease blood pressure and reduce overall levels of tension.

Although alcohol is the most commonly used and abused depressant, and is certainly an addictive drug that causes harm, this book will focus on drugs besides alcohol. If you're interested in exploring the issues specific to alcohol use, you may want to check out another book in The Almost Effect series, *Almost Alcoholic*, by Robert Doyle, MD, and Joseph Nowinski, PhD.

Most other depressants usually come in pill form, with heroin as a notable exception, and can be used for medical reasons when prescribed by physicians. Major subgroups of depressants include opiate painkillers and benzodiazepines.

Opiate medications are all either naturally based or synthetically produced cousins of heroin. This category includes OxyContin, Vicodin, and Percocet. They work well for relieving pain, and for many people they produce calm, warm, euphoric feelings. Indeed, many people with opiate addiction become almost wistful as they recount the complete, total sense of well-being and calm they felt upon first using opiates. (Inevitably, however, they never achieve this same state again and, because of changes in brain chemistry, begin taking the drug just to feel normal and to avoid the horrible feelings of withdrawal.)

The other broad category of depressants is benzodiazepines, or benzos. Benzos are terrific for relieving anxiety, especially in the short term. They can also help people fall asleep. Among the more commonly used (and abused) benzos are Valium, Klonopin, Ativan, and Xanax.

Although depressant medications can produce helpful medical effects in the short term, they can cause confusion, lethargy, and disorientation in people who abuse them. Prolonged use is quite dangerous because it can easily produce physical dependence. Even after just several weeks of using depressants, users can build tolerance, and their bodies scream out in distress when they stop taking them.

Hallucinogens

Hallucinogens are the third major category of commonly abused drugs. Hallucinogens include LSD (lysergic acid diethylamide), mushrooms (psilocybin), mescaline, and Salvia (Salvia divinorum). The appeal of hallucinogens lies in their ability to produce—as their name suggests—significant hallucinations, visions, and dream states. Some people claim that taking these kinds of drugs causes them to think more clearly and deeply about important matters.

As such, individuals who are under the influence of hallucinogens can behave quite erratically and potentially very dangerously because their normal judgment is essentially shut off while they are under the influence. Moreover, some hallucinogens, potentially LSD and certainly Salvia and PCP (phencyclidine, also known as angel dust), can produce terrifying images and visions and cause substantial distress while users are high. Coming down from the high can also be tricky. Often, users report feeling "strange" and "out of it" in the period after being high. Regular use can bring prolonged uneasiness or hallucinations, even long after the drug has left one's body, and is known to bring on chronic psychosis in vulnerable individuals.

Marijuana

Marijuana is really in a class by itself. Unlike the drugs discussed above that are fairly easy to group into one category or another, marijuana defies simple categorization and actually has properties of each of the above categories. It can be stimulating for many individuals, it can be calming and soothing for others, and for some it can even be hallucinogenic. Regardless of how you categorize it, marijuana is by far the most commonly used drug, aside from alcohol.

The complexity of marijuana doesn't just stop with its myriad effects on one's mental state. One also needs to consider the use of medical marijuana. Marijuana can be helpful in increasing appetite, reducing pain, alleviating nausea (common among people undergoing chemotherapy), decreasing intraocular (inside the eye) pressure in people with glaucoma, and helping reduce some symptoms of certain neurological disorders. In these instances, its use should be supported when prescribed by a competent health care professional. However, much of what is prescribed as medical marijuana—in locales where it is permitted—is little more than a legal way of obtaining marijuana for illicit purposes. For example, when I've been jogging on the boardwalk in Venice Beach in California, I've been asked—even as I was running by—numerous times to stop and come into medical marijuana dispensaries and obtain marijuana on the spot, usually with an enticement such as "The doctor is in." We'd be hard-pressed to say that in those instances the marijuana being prescribed was for any legitimate medical purpose.

• • •

I decided to write this book so that people who are almost addicted to these drugs—or in many cases their concerned loved ones—would have a guidebook for sorting through the many questions and issues that arise from the drug use, including these in particular:

1. How can people who are almost addicted find some clarity about their drug use and decide whether they've arrived at the time when they need to make a change?

2. How can family members determine whether or not their loved one has crossed into the almost addicted realm?

3. For those who *do* decide that their drug use—or a loved one's drug use—has crossed into almost addicted territory, how should they proceed and what resources are available to them?

These are important questions, especially because people who are almost addicted usually don't think they need to change anything about how they use drugs. After all, they can reassure themselves that their substance use is not problematic because, as far as they can tell, it has never caused harm in any area of their lives. They have never lost a job because of their drug use. Indeed, they are repeatedly praised for being a great worker and just won a promotion! Their children are doing fine in school! They have never been arrested! What's the problem? Why don't you quit bothering them and go help one of those people with a *true* addiction?

If that's not enough proof, they also feel fit and healthy—in fact, at their last checkup, their primary care physician gave them a clean bill of health. This last point is important for readers who are almost addicted: when these individuals present themselves to a primary care doctor, a psychiatrist, or any other medical professional, they only rarely cite substance use as a problem for themselves. Far more often, they will complain of problems like anxiety, an inability to focus or pay attention, trouble sleeping, or low mood. In short, *almost* addiction can cause very real problems, even if they're not obvious to the person involved.

Who This Book Is For

This book can help readers who are almost addicted—and their family members—determine whether a problem is brewing. It will also help point them toward solutions and answers. This sort of manual is particularly important for people who are almost addicted, who may fly below the radar of many health care professionals, since their lives are not in utter chaos or ruin from their substance use. After all, when they have a patient's full story, psychiatrists and primary care physicians rarely miss diagnosing a true addiction, but it is fairly easy for a physician either to entirely miss the symptoms in those with almost addiction or to choose to ignore their problem. Given the ever-tightening constraints on the time that we physicians can spend with patients, this problem identifying almost addicted patients will likely continue to get worse.

That is why an awareness of almost addiction is more important than ever. Individuals (and their family members) need to be able to spot a problem before it creates chaos and to see and evaluate their own relationship to substances as clearly as possible. If you're almost addicted, or you have someone in your life who is almost addicted, you are suffering from a problem that does not have to be occurring. This book can help end that suffering.

Now is the time to sort through whether or not you or someone you care about is almost addicted. If so, it's time to learn how to take steps to minimize the harmful effects of drug use and help yourself—or the almost addicted person you're trying to help—find a better life.

This book will begin by showing you how people become almost addicted and then describe how they think, feel, and behave when they're almost addicted. You'll also learn numerous methods of initiating a change for the better.

Change is never easy, and it is especially hard for people who are even partly under the grip of an intoxicating substance. Nevertheless, modifying the behaviors of people who are almost addicted is certainly possible, and it can bring about dramatic improvements in the overall quality of life not only for the individuals themselves but for those around them.

■ ◆ ■

Part 1

A Problem Emerges
from the Shadows

1

Almost Addiction,
but Very Much a Concern

Although I could talk at length about what the almost addicted individual looks like from a psychiatrist's perspective, it may be more helpful for you to read some accounts of the various types of real-life situations I've encountered with patients over the years.

If you're unsure whether your drug use has reached the level of almost addiction—or if a loved one could fall into this category—consider whether you identify with the person you'll meet in each chapter. The people depicted here are composites with identifying details changed; none of them represents a single real person. But the causes and consequences of their almost addiction are true-to-life examples of how this problem can arise and harm people's lives.

Bridget's Story

When Bridget came to see me for the first time, she had recently visited her primary care physician for a regular checkup. At the visit, she had told her doctor that she was depressed, anxious, and in desperate need of relief, so he referred her to my office.

Bridget, who was thirty years old and working as a restaurant manager when we met, grew up in central New Jersey. Between the ages of five and seven, she was sexually abused by a teenage neighbor. She tearfully told me that she didn't tell anyone about it until many years later because the boy had threatened to kill her family's dog if she told.

Bridget had a good relationship with her father until she was thirteen, when he left the family and moved to a nearby town. After that, they only had infrequent contact. Her mother was devastated by his departure and the subsequent divorce, and she began neglecting her household duties. Bridget stepped up to keep the home functioning. She recalled that this is when she learned to hold in her emotions.

After high school, Bridget moved to a neighboring state for college. To support herself while attending school, she began working as a restaurant hostess. When a serving position opened up, she began waiting tables, much to her delight, because it paid much better than hosting. Drug use was rampant at the restaurant, with the cooks and the restaurant manager preferring cocaine as the drug of choice. During the time she worked there, Bridget tried cocaine twice.

Although she was a decent student majoring in business, she dropped out at the end of her sophomore year, partly due to her first episode of depression, which was related to emerging memories of the sexual abuse she'd previously repressed.

When Bridget came to see me, she was experiencing another episode of major depression along with considerable panic and anxiety. Her symptoms—including poor sleep, loss of interest in activities she previously enjoyed, increased appetite, and occasional feelings of wanting to be dead—had gone on for months. Her panic attacks came almost every day, with sweating, heart palpitations, shortness of breath, and a sense that she was going to die. I eventually learned that depression and anxiety were common in both of her parents' families.

She attributed her symptoms almost entirely to difficulties she was having in a year-long relationship. Although she said she loved her boyfriend—and the sex was the best she'd ever had—he was so jealous and controlling that she couldn't go out alone without him becoming irate. She also suspected that he was seeing other women.

She knew she needed to leave him and routinely asked herself why she stayed. Even more than the sex, she didn't want to walk away because she was tired of her relationships failing and wanted one to succeed. Specifically, she "didn't want to feel like a loser again."

Nowhere in his referral did the primary care doctor mention substance use. When meeting with new patients, I always try to ask about drug use (I say "try" because in certain situations, like flagrant psychosis or raging mania, doing this can be impossible). At our first meeting, Bridget was very forthcoming about her drug use. She said that over the previous six months, she'd ramped up her marijuana use to smoking a joint three to four evenings a week. Bridget said marijuana helped her to relax and cope with the stress from her relationship.

In addition to using marijuana, she was snorting cocaine

regularly. She said that although she was previously using cocaine once a year—which seemed like relatively light use compared to many of her restaurant co-workers—over the last six months she'd been using cocaine every other week. She said it provided her with a "means of escape."

When I asked if the marijuana and cocaine caused any problems in her life, Bridget couldn't think of any. She simply thought that these drugs helped her relax, feel good, and escape the stress of her daily life—and that as far as she could tell, neither had any adverse effects on her.

Although I didn't want to begin our working relationship by correcting her or making her feel any worse than she already felt, I gently explained that the drug use might in fact be *contributing* to her symptoms of depression, anxiety, and panic. After all, it only makes sense that her drug use would factor into the symptoms. To illustrate why, I like to think about Isaac Newton's third law of motion, which states that *for every action there is an equal and opposite reaction.* Loosely applied to drug use, this law suggests that if the immediate effect of marijuana is to cause people to feel relaxed and calm, then as the drug leaves the body and immediately thereafter, the equal and opposite reaction occurs and they feel more anxious and hyped up, whether or not they are even aware of it. Conversely, if cocaine's immediate effect is to excite, stimulate, and thrill, when it leaves the body, the person may feel emptied out and depressed.

So, although Bridget didn't see any connection between her drug use and her symptoms when she walked through my door, the drugs very well could have been contributing to her symptoms of depression, panic, and anxiety.

How *Almost* Addiction Differs from *True* Addiction

To better understand almost addiction, it's important to first understand what constitutes true addiction, or *dependence*. Once you know that, you can get a good grasp on the ways in which Bridget's drug use does *not* meet the definition of addiction.

Several features are essential for establishing that people have a true dependence on substances like marijuana, cocaine, and opiates. Looking at these symptoms one by one will help you to see the line between full-blown addiction and being almost addicted.

Someone who is truly addicted to a drug shows

- tolerance
- withdrawal
- loss of control when it comes to the drug
- inability to stop using the drug
- obsession or preoccupation with obtaining and using the drug

Tolerance

Let's start by understanding *tolerance*, one of the essential ingredients in addiction. Tolerance means that when someone is addicted, any given amount of the drug packs less of a punch than it previously did. As a result, people with addiction require ever-increasing amounts of their drug in order to get high.

This phenomenon is seen in those who drink alcohol daily, even in moderation. As the months and years wear on, these drinkers usually need more alcohol to achieve the same "buzz" as before. Similarly, opiate addiction often spurs users to escalate their intake dramatically over time to try to achieve the same high they used to enjoy. One patient I worked with went from using 20 to 40 milligrams of OxyContin each day to more than 900 milligrams daily in the span of just a year and a half. Still, no one around him, including his wife, even suspected that something was wrong—and he was taking a daily dose that would be large enough to kill a group of more than five people who were new to the drug.

For people with opiate addiction in particular, tolerance can have severe consequences. First, because of their cost when obtained illegally, opiate medications can quickly become prohibitively expensive. When users can no longer afford their drug of choice, many of them turn to heroin because it produces the same high at a much lower cost. This is a problem, because injecting drugs (which many people who use heroin will ultimately resort to doing) poses a whole new level of health risks. Second, since tolerance dwindles when a person stops using opiates, addicted individuals who have been clean for some time and then relapse are prone to overdose and die if they immediately resume using the same dose they last used.

Withdrawal

A second feature of addiction is that the individual experiences *withdrawal* when the drug is leaving the body. Withdrawal is often very uncomfortable physically and emotionally, although its precise nature varies depending on the drug. Inevitably, people with addictions relieve their withdrawal by using more of the drug, which of course only reinforces the addiction. For most drugs that are abused, including opiates and benzodiazepines, the effects of withdrawal can be tremendously unpleasant. In rare instances, withdrawal can cause seizures or death.

Although almost anyone who watches television or movies (much less anyone who knows someone addicted to opiates or alcohol) has an idea what withdrawal may look like, many assume that marijuana causes no withdrawal effects. Even a lot of pot smokers say that they never experience withdrawal symptoms. Science, however, begs to differ. Emerging research is showing that withdrawal symptoms from marijuana *do* indeed exist. For example, one 2011 study found that when frequent users abruptly stop marijuana use, their blood pressure rises.[8] In some people who smoke marijuana, the rise may be quite substantial. A 2010 study found that 42 percent of cannabis users had experienced withdrawal symptoms. Common symptoms included craving the drug, trouble falling asleep, sadness, nervousness, irritability, and headaches. (On the plus side, many reported improved memory after stopping use.)[9]

Loss of Control

Another feature of addiction is that of *losing control* over the substance, so users end up using more or for a longer period of time than planned. Although this book is focused on drugs other than alcohol, readers may have witnessed this loss of control in people who can't stop after a couple of drinks. (One of my Irish American patients calls this the Irish curse: "One drink is too many and ten is not enough.") This is also evident in the individual who snorts cocaine uncontrollably and then gets into fights and winds up arrested for assault.

Inability to Stop Using

Another criterion of addiction is an *inability to stop* using the drug, which means that the person has repeatedly failed attempts to stop or cut down. People with true addiction continue using their drugs even though they know that physical or psychological problems may result. Ask people with a heroin addiction how the drug has caused them harm and they can almost always reel off a long list of very serious problems connected to their use. Yet this knowledge doesn't deter them from doing anything possible to obtain their next fix.

Obsession

Another aspect of addiction is that the individual *spends a lot of time* obtaining the drug, thinking about the drug, or using the drug. Individuals addicted to heroin, for example, may say that heroin is on their minds *all* of the time, day in and day out, and that they will do just about anything to ensure they don't run out—including lying, stealing, cheating, and having sex for money. Similarly, people addicted to marijuana often spend inordinate amounts of time thinking about pot, smoking it, and discussing it with friends.

Considering these five criteria, you can see that Bridget is clearly *not* addicted to marijuana or cocaine. She smokes pot regularly but not every day. She has gone days without either drug and not experienced any withdrawal symptoms. And her life does not revolve around marijuana and coke. She doesn't spend much time obtaining them because she knows who to call, and she does so infrequently. Furthermore, she has never lost control of her drug use. Nobody around her, such as her friends and neighbors, would suspect that she uses. She's never been arrested for drugs nor has she appeared on her town's crime blotter.

How Almost Addiction Differs from Substance Abuse

We've just examined the criteria for substance dependence, and Bridget clearly does not meet them. But could you say that she is a substance *abuser* instead? To meet the official criteria for substance abuse, the person needs to have significant impairment or distress as a result of maladaptive (meaning unhealthy) substance use that is recurring over a twelve-month period, with at least one of the following criteria:

- Failure to fulfill major obligations at home, school, or work, for example, repeated absences or poor performance as a result of substance use
- Repeated instances of using substances when doing so is potentially physically hazardous, for example, driving or using heavy machinery while high
- Recurrent legal problems as a result of substance use
- Continued use despite having persistent or recurrent social or interpersonal problems

There are several key differences between substance dependence and substance abuse. People who are substance *abusers* aren't fixated on the drug like someone who is dependent, they haven't developed physical dependence on it, and they don't experience withdrawal symptoms when deprived of it.

It's important to note that, as I write this, a revision is underway for the diagnostic manual for psychiatry, the *Diagnostic and Statistical Manual of Mental Disorders*, fourth edition, text revision *(DSM-IV-TR)*. Its authors recognize that these two categories—dependence and abuse—are too rigidly defined and don't acknowledge the full spectrum of drug use that spans recreational, nonproblematic use all the way to full-blown dependence. Just as I am recommending that addiction be viewed on a continuum, the professionals behind the forthcoming fifth edition *(DSM-V)* are arriving at the same conclusion. While working on the manual, they have proposed a single diagnosis, "substance use disorder," with one qualifier being "moderate" and the other being "severe."

What does this planned change mean? It means that the best minds in psychiatry see substance use as occurring on a spectrum and that the current categories of diagnosis do not suffice. Furthermore, the planned changes for the *DSM* endorse the idea that a level of problematic substance use exists that falls below levels that are diagnosable. People at this level are those I am calling *almost addicted*, a group that included Bridget.

The Drug-Using World

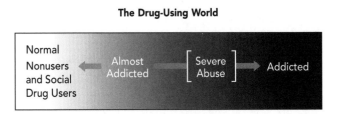

The critical difference between the way I see the drug-using world and the traditional view of drug use is shown by the shading from white to a gray that grows darker until it becomes black, creating the zones shown in this graphic. The large gray area (where Bridget is now) separates the white zone of what experts would call normal nonuse or occasional social drug use from the black zone of true addiction.

How Do I Identify Someone Who Is Almost Addicted?

Having ruled out what almost addiction *isn't*, I can define what it *is*. For drug use to meet the criteria of almost addiction, it must

- fall outside what is regarded as normal behavior, but come short of meeting traditional *DSM* criteria for a diagnosable disorder

- currently cause problems for the person or for loved ones or other bystanders

- have the potential to progress to a diagnosis of drug abuse or drug dependence, but even if it doesn't, it can still cause substantial problems

A final characteristic is that addressing almost addiction may improve the health or quality of life for the individual or others around him.

As mentioned in the foreword, in recent years, experts in many medical fields have been focusing more attention on other "almost" problems, though in some cases these are called *pre*-problems. These include prediabetes, pre-hypertension, and levels of cholesterol that previously weren't defined as a concern. Prediabetes puts people at higher risk of having full-blown diabetes. Pre-hypertension makes people more likely to develop high blood pressure. And in the meantime, these problems can cause physical damage even if they don't progress to the "real" thing.

As a result, almost addiction falls easily into the increasingly accepted category of problems that need to be recognized and treated much earlier than they have been in the past. A number of screening tools are available to sort out whether someone might have a diagnosable substance-related disorder (or fall short of having a diagnosable condition). One of the easiest to use is the Drug Abuse Screening Test (DAST).[10] The DAST-20 version consists of twenty yes-or-no questions. To tally your score, give yourself one point for each "yes" answer—except for questions 4 and 5: for those, give yourself one point for each "no" answer.

A score of 6 or more indicates a likely diagnosis of substance abuse or dependence. The almost addicted category, on the other hand, will include people with scores of 1 through 5. However, since no screening tool is perfect, some people who are almost addicted may also score 6 or more. It's a quick way of gauging whether you or someone you care about may be almost addicted.

Drug Abuse Screening Test (DAST)

1. Have you used drugs other than those required for medical reasons?
   ☐ YES ☐ NO

2. Have you abused prescription drugs?
   ☐ YES ☐ NO

3. Do you abuse more than one drug at a time?
   ☐ YES ☐ NO

4. Can you get through the week without using drugs?
   ☐ YES ☐ NO

5. Are you always able to stop using drugs when you want to?
   ☐ YES ☐ NO

6. Have you had "blackouts" or "flashbacks" as a result of drug use?
   ☐ YES ☐ NO

7. Do you ever feel bad or guilty about your drug use?
   ☐ YES   ☐ NO

8. Does your spouse (or parents) ever complain about your involvement with drugs?
   ☐ YES   ☐ NO

9. Has drug abuse created problems between you and your spouse or your parents?
   ☐ YES   ☐ NO

10. Have you lost friends because of your use of drugs?
    ☐ YES   ☐ NO

11. Have you neglected your family because of your use of drugs?
    ☐ YES   ☐ NO

12. Have you been in trouble at work because of your use of drugs?
    ☐ YES   ☐ NO

13. Have you lost a job because of drug abuse?
    ☐ YES   ☐ NO

14. Have you gotten into fights when under the influence of drugs?
    ☐ YES   ☐ NO

15. Have you engaged in illegal activities in order to obtain drugs?
    ☐ YES   ☐ NO

16. Have you been arrested for possession of illegal drugs?
    ☐ YES   ☐ NO

QUIZ CONTINUED ON NEXT PAGE

17. Have you ever experienced withdrawal symptoms (felt sick) when you stopped taking a drug?

    ☐ YES   ☐ NO

18. Have you had medical problems as a result of your drug use (e.g., memory loss, hepatitis, convulsions, bleeding, etc.)?

    ☐ YES   ☐ NO

19. Have you gone to anyone for help for a drug problem?

    ☐ YES   ☐ NO

20. Have you been involved in a treatment program especially related to drug use?

    ☐ YES   ☐ NO

YOUR TOTAL SCORE: _____ Yes   _____ No

For questions 4 and 5, give yourself one point for each "no" answer.
For all other questions, give yourself one point for each "yes" answer.

Bridget would probably answer yes to just three of these questions: She has used drugs other than those required for medical reasons, she uses more than one drug, and she has engaged in illegal activities to obtain them (buying marijuana and cocaine is against the law). It's also possible that she would have trouble getting through the week without using marijuana, since she smokes it several nights a week. However, her boyfriend has never objected to her drug use, and her answers to the rest of the questions on the DAST would not raise red flags.

But although Bridget is not addicted to drugs and doesn't meet the criteria for drug abuse, her cocaine use has a large effect on her life. She knows it's illegal, so she always uses it with some trepidation. She has to double-check her luggage any time she travels to ensure she's not carrying any cocaine.

Getting high from cocaine and marijuana probably also allowed Bridget to check out of her life just enough so she could avoid looking too deeply within. If she'd been focused enough to take a closer look at herself, she might have found the need to make some big changes in her life, such as leaving her boyfriend earlier or delving into her history of sexual abuse so she might be able to put it behind her. After she finally parted ways with her boyfriend, Bridget realized that her on-going drug use was keeping her tied to her past, since she had leaned on drugs more heavily as she endured more and more of her boyfriend's emotional abuse.

Although she initially denied any connection, the amount of marijuana and cocaine Bridget was using likely made her mood worse. Over the long term, marijuana is a depressant. And cocaine, with its ability to ramp up anxiety while users are high and then send them crashing into lethargy and depression afterward, was clearly not helping her situation, despite her infrequent use.

As someone who was almost addicted, Bridget had a lot of company. Over the years, I have seen many individuals whose substance use, though nondependent, created many psychiatric difficulties. I have seen patients prone to panic and anxiety experience full-blown panic attacks—with symptoms that included sweating, heart palpitations, shortness of breath, and a sense of impending doom—when the single benzodiazepine tranquilizer they took recreationally was wearing off. I have seen people become completely psychotic, with paranoia, delusions, and visual hallucinations, after smoking just a small amount of marijuana. In one case, the cannabis-induced psychosis lasted several weeks. (Fortunately this person hasn't touched marijuana in the decade since this unpleasant event.)

Since almost addiction is such an underrecognized problem, the idea that occasional drug use could be harming your life may be a totally new concept to you. Even your doctor may scratch her head for a moment while she absorbs what it might mean for a patient to have a drug problem but not be quite addicted.

As a result, in addition to filling out the DAST, I'd like you to ask yourself whether you (or your loved one) may be seeing these other issues as well:

- While out with friends, do you frequently use more drugs than you'd planned?
- Do you prefer smoking marijuana to socializing with friends who don't smoke?
- Does your drug use isolate you from others?
- Have you damaged important relationships in your life because of your drug use?
- After a night of partying and taking cocaine or some other drug, have you slept with someone you shouldn't have?
- While under the influence, have you signed a contract that you wouldn't otherwise have agreed to?
- Do you find yourself daydreaming about when you can get high again?

- Have you gotten angry when someone has confronted you about your drug use?
- Have you committed a crime while under the influence?
- Have you given up activities you used to enjoy?
- Are you forgetful?
- Are money or other valuable objects disappearing from around the house?
- Are you failing to show up for important functions?
- Are you evasive in answering questions about where you've been or who you were with?
- Are you taking more risks than usual?
- Are you failing to attend to your appearance as usual?

If you answer yes to more than one or two of these questions, this adds to the evidence that you (or your loved one) may be almost addicted.

Almost Addicted No More: The First Steps to Take

Later in the book, you'll find an entire section devoted to helping people cope when a friend or loved one is almost addicted, and another section aimed at helping almost addicted readers confront their own problem. However, if your responses to the DAST test or the other questions point to almost addiction, you don't have to wait—taking just a few small steps now will help you begin the journey away from drug use. If you believe you may be almost addicted, consider taking the following suggestions.

If you're reading this book on behalf of someone you care about who may be almost addicted, this advice may be helpful in getting the individual to become aware of the problem, which is an important first step. However, I recommend reading part 3—which is directed at friends and loved ones of people who are almost addicted—before approaching the individual with any recommendations from this book.

Consider the Implications of Your Answers

If your answers to the questions earlier in this chapter suggest you're almost addicted, how does that make you feel? Do you agree that you may have a drug problem? Or do you feel defensive or angry at the suggestion? Are you ready to cut back on your drug use or even stop it altogether? If not, can you see yourself cutting back or quitting in the future?

Think about Your History of Drug Use

If your responses suggest that you're almost addicted, think back to when you first smoked marijuana or started using other drugs. What made you decide to start? What was going on in your life at the time that may have played a role in launching your drug use? Like Bridget's experience, could drug use have been a way to self-medicate to deal with unhappy events from your childhood?

While growing up, what examples of drug use did you see from family members, friends, and other important people in your life? If they used drugs, did their substance use play any role in your practices?

What Would Keep You from Stopping Now?

If you realized that you had to stop using your drug of choice for any reason, what factors might make quitting difficult or uncomfortable? Would anxiety over some aspect of your life or your past increase if you couldn't use? Would you have trouble remaining in your circle of friends if you were no longer using?

Would you lose a part of your identity that is important to you? Would walking away from the drug feel like you were cutting out an important part of your daily routine?

What Would You Gain from Stopping Now?

Similarly, ask yourself what positive changes might arise if you stopped using this drug.

- Would you have more money to spend on necessities or luxuries?

- Would you have more time to devote to hobbies?

- Would you benefit from better mental focus?

- Would you do better at work?

- Would you have a better relationship with your family?

- Would you be in a better position to resolve painful events from your past rather than trying to deal with them through drugs?

- Would any anxiety and depression you experience improve if you were to quit using drugs or to use only infrequently? (The answer to this question is almost always yes.)

- Is it possible that your drug use has a more harmful effect than you care to acknowledge?

Answering the above questions about yourself, or asking a loved one to answer them, can be very difficult because these issues may be painful to consider. Also, most people are remarkably skilled at not seeing themselves or their loved ones clearly. This is why physicians are advised to never treat themselves or their family members, since their judgments about someone close to them can be clouded.

The kind of understanding and awareness necessary to honestly answer these questions takes time to develop, so hang in there and keep gathering more information to help you determine whether you (or a loved one) would benefit from a change.

Bridget's Outcome

I worked with Bridget for about four years, seeing her every two to four weeks during rough times and every three to four months when her life was going well. I never wavered in my stance that her substance use was not helping her emotional issues and was likely making matters worse. Although I initially treaded lightly, over time—when we had learned to trust and respect each other—I was able to be more direct.

Since her symptoms of depression and anxiety were substantial and nearly debilitating, I initially focused on finding medication options to help her feel better. I prescribed an antidepressant, knowing that these medications can help with both depression and anxiety. Bridget did begin to feel some relief with the antidepressant, and she eventually felt strong enough to finally leave her relationship.

At our last visit before she moved away, Bridget had been completely clean from marijuana and cocaine for a year and a half. She was also almost weaned off her antidepressant medication and poised to completely stop it soon. Of course, she could have a recurrence of depression someday, especially since she has a history of trauma and a family history of depression. But for the time being, she was healthy and well and not further complicating her life and her mental state by using drugs.

■ ◆ ■

2

Why Should I Change?

Many substance users who meet the definition of almost addiction see no reason why they should stop using drugs. Because the harmful effects of being almost addicted don't always scream out like the often obvious effects of true addiction, users may feel little pressure or incentive to stop or even alter their relationship with drugs. Of course, many people are motivated to quit using simply because most of these drugs are illegal. Users are not only breaking the law and risking arrest and legal problems, they are also supporting a supply chain of dealers and traffickers who are often tied to criminal organizations such as the drug lords and cartels who harm and even kill people in the course of doing business.

But, legal and ethical issues aside, the physical and psychological damage caused by drug use for the almost addicted is quite real, even if it doesn't always raise red flags and alarms. To see how another real person suffered from almost addiction, let's consider the case of Mike.

Mike's Story

Mike was in his late thirties when he came to see me. He wasn't thrilled to be in my office; his wife had insisted he come in after he was arrested for driving under the influence (DUI). To his neighbors, Mike would look like one of society's winners. He was a top-level executive at an investment bank and lived in a multimillion-dollar home in one of the nicest suburbs of his city. He was trim, fit, and handsome.

Although Mike was a bit reserved, over the eight months we worked together, he gradually opened up and told me his life story. He had a happy, uneventful childhood. His father owned a hardware store and his mother was an elementary school teacher. In high school, he was captain of the varsity tennis team and was a solid B student. After high school, he studied economics at a mid-tier college.

Shortly after college, he began working for a major investment bank and quickly developed a knack for understanding trends and market forces. With his natural skills, drive to succeed, and a few lucky breaks, he soon made a name for himself as an up-and-comer. His job titles steadily grew more impressive.

Mike was married to Janine, a woman his age who had also known a lot of success in her career. But after their child was born, his wife decided to take a break from the corporate world to be a full-time mother. What they'd initially planned as a short-term hiatus became a new life for Janine when she decided she would be happier and healthier staying home for good.

After Janine pulled out of the workforce, the couple began to grow apart. Her new life revolved around the day-to-day activities of caring for their child and tending to their household, while Mike's world centered on helping his bank prosper.

He worked long hours—it was always difficult just to schedule our office visits—and traveled often. He had trouble finding room in his calendar for face time with Janine.

That's the image his co-workers saw. What they didn't see was the drug use in Mike's life. Mike started smoking pot in high school and continued into adulthood. When he came to see me, he was smoking once or twice a week. He said marijuana wasn't something he relied on to cope with stress but, instead, was just something that made him feel good. He didn't think his pot use was problematic at all, except for the fact that it's illegal in most parts of the United States.

Mike did acknowledge that his wife did not approve of marijuana, that she had asked him to quit more than once, and that she was worried about what would happen if the authorities ever found marijuana on him. So he did not keep pot at home and only smoked when he was away from Janine.

By the time I met him, Mike would drink socially with friends or when out in the evening at business functions, but he rarely drank during the week. Apart from the DUI arrest that brought him to my office, he'd never felt guilty about either his drinking or his marijuana smoking, and he'd never been arrested before.

I also learned that Mike was having an affair with Ana, an executive in a company his bank worked with. She was attractive, adventurous, intelligent, and loved spending any time she could with Mike, which usually amounted to a couple of times per month, often when he was traveling for work. In the evenings when they were together, Mike and Ana often smoked marijuana.

On the night of his arrest, Mike had been out with a couple

of close friends at dinner and then headed to a nightclub afterward. At dinner he had a couple of drinks, and at the club he had two more. During the evening, he also smoked half a marijuana joint. When he headed home, he said he felt a bit of a buzz, but did not feel intoxicated or unsafe.

Mike was almost home when a car in front of him suddenly stopped to avoid hitting an animal in the road. Mike rear-ended the car. Fortunately, neither driver was injured, but when the police arrived, they asked Mike several questions, including whether he'd had anything to drink prior to the accident.

Mike answered truthfully and was then asked to blow into a Breathalyzer device. He refused. He assumed, erroneously, that the device would detect the marijuana in his system. Regardless, since he'd had five drinks in the previous eight hours—a heavy night for him—his blood alcohol level might have been above the legal limit.

Although he didn't take the Breathalyzer test, Mike failed the field sobriety test he was administered and was arrested and charged with driving under the influence. When I met with him, Mike's driving privileges had been suspended and he was forced to take public transportation to work and elsewhere. (Mike didn't know it, but in the state where he lived, his refusal to take the Breathalyzer test made him ineligible for a "hardship license" to drive to and from work while his case was being decided.)

Although he pleaded not guilty and hired a lawyer to fight the DUI charges, he found himself awaiting a court decision that could cost him thousands of dollars and theoretically land him in jail. He wondered what would happen if the news of his arrest hit the papers. What if his partners in the firm learned of his encounter with the law? He'd made more than a few enemies in the workplace over the years and he wondered if they'd use this against him. If word got out, would he be demoted—or even drummed out of the firm?

When the Consequences of Almost Addiction Hit Home

Those who knew him, including myself, would never think that Mike was addicted to either alcohol or marijuana. Other than the charge of driving under the influence, which was the reason he came into my office, Mike had never been in any trouble because of his substance use. He was steadily employed (and making more than half a million a year), had a family, and owned a home. And yet the sum total of his marijuana and alcohol use strongly suggested that he was almost addicted.

If Mike took the DAST test included in the last chapter—which gives people a sense of whether drug use is a problem in their lives—he would likely have a score of 4, adding weight to the likelihood that he's almost addicted.

For people who are substance abusers, and especially for those who are dependent on substances (which is an even higher level of concern), the costs of drug use are often obvious and devastating. These costs include empty bank accounts, criminal charges, pummeled relationships, damaged health, and various other personal losses. However, people who are almost addicted can also experience these same outcomes.

The repercussions of drug use can hit hard, swiftly, and without warning, even if you've been using drugs occasionally for years without problems. The cost of almost addiction may come in various forms.

Employment and Financial Costs

The economic toll of illicit drug use is staggeringly high, and the activities of people who are almost addicted account for a substantial portion of this cost. Although many people who are almost addicted are employed and doing well in their jobs, problem-causing substance use decreases people's chances of either finding or holding on to a job, according to a 2011 German study that reviewed research findings from the past twenty years.[11] This same study also found that the relationship between substance use and job troubles also goes the other way. That is, being unemployed is a significant risk factor for drug use—and for developing substance-related disorders.

Another study, from 2009, found a significant and direct relationship between higher unemployment rates in a given geographic area and higher rate of opiate use.[12] Both of these studies suggest that drug use causes a spectrum of work disruption, so that even people whose drug use does not rise to the abuse or dependence level are more likely to have problems at work.

Let's go back to Mike. Before his DUI arrest, he had not experienced any problems at work directly related to his alcohol or marijuana use, yet his marijuana use did pose a number of potential threats to his lifestyle. If you're using drugs, they could threaten the way you live your life, as well.

The first threat stems from the simple fact that where Mike lives, marijuana is illegal and, as such, every time he buys it or smokes it he is taking a risk. You may think that to be arrested for marijuana—at least in most places in the United States—you'd have to be fairly blatant or careless about lighting up in some way. But even discreet use of pot purchased from a well-known supplier carries the risk of arrest and accompanying public shame and possible loss of employment.

Think that no one would ever arrest you for possessing or using marijuana? In 2009, police made more than 1.6 million arrests in the United States for drug violations. About 46 percent of these were for marijuana possession.[13] In Europe, reported drug law offenses rose from the mid-1990s to 2008.[14]

A drug arrest can become more than an embarrassment. It could be a little snowball that grows as it crashes through your life. Were Mike ever to be arrested on illicit drug charges, it would take only a small group of disgruntled co-workers in his office to create a ruckus that would jeopardize his job.

How about you? If you live in a small town or a midsize city, how would your employers react if your name showed up in the newspaper after a drug arrest? Would they be understanding? Would they give you a second chance? After years of suffering through high unemployment, layoffs, and tight job markets, most workers are acutely aware that any misstep affecting their reputation at work could lead to a long stretch without a job.

Separately, although Mike's relationship with his mistress was not based on their mutual attraction to pot, smoking marijuana together certainly had become a staple in their relationship. Over the years, I have come to see that when secret relationships are going smoothly—like the affair Mike was having—nobody calls the police or notifies the spouse about what's happening behind closed doors. However, once a relationship ends (and I hate to break the news to the optimists out there, but with very few exceptions nearly every romantic relationship ends prior to your death), all bets are off about who's going to say what to whom.

What's the risk here? If Mike ultimately doesn't leave his wife, Janine, for his mistress, Ana, and Ana eventually gets tired of waiting—as mistresses often do—she might be peeved enough to inform Mike's colleagues about the times that she's seen him take work calls after smoking pot or about the deals that were struck between her company and Mike's while they were having their affair. Mike would have to be supremely naive to believe that his marijuana use wasn't jeopardizing his job.

But that's Mike's story. If you are using substances, you may still be wondering how your drug use could affect you. What if you got busted with pot—or meth, cocaine, LSD, heroin, or unprescribed OxyContin—in your system? Even if you did manage to keep your job initially, what kind of lawyer could you afford? (Would it be a well-connected, hard-working lawyer like the one Mike could arrange, or would you have to settle for less?)

Do you have time in your work schedule to make the court appearances and probation visits you may suddenly have to keep? Could you lose any work-related licenses or certifications? If you lose your driving privileges, who's going to bring you to work? When the next round of promotions comes up, will your bosses want to move you up the ladder? Or will they choose the person who wasn't arrested for drug use, if all other factors are equal?

Each toke you inhale, each line of coke you snort, and each hit of Ecstasy you swallow could be the one that brings your career to a screeching halt. If you tell yourself afterward, "Well, at least I'm not an addict," is that going to bring you much comfort? It's certainly not going to pay your bills.

Another Threat from Drug Use: Human Resources

If the human resources department in Mike's company had learned of his behaviors, he likely would have faced serious repercussions. To illustrate, here's the drug and alcohol policy from Harvard University's HR department as of 2012. Mike wasn't a Harvard employee. However, having perused a number of such policies, I think this one seems fairly typical:

> Violations of laws relating to controlled substances or alcohol are prohibited on Harvard premises, in vehicles provided by Harvard, at any work site or location at which University duties are being performed by Harvard staff members, or as part of any other Harvard activities.
>
> Employees may not manufacture, use, distribute, or dispense controlled substances in the workplace.
>
> Common examples of controlled substances, as defined by law, are cocaine, marijuana, and heroin.
>
> The University will take disciplinary action against violators. Such disciplinary action may include:
>
> - satisfactory participation in a substance abuse treatment, counseling or education program,
> - suspension,
> - termination of employment and referral for prosecution[15]

This policy applies not only on Harvard premises but anywhere an employee is performing work duties. So if Mike uses illicit drugs while on company business, he is violating the rules set up by most HR departments and risking his job. Mike was taking a chance by having an intimate relationship with a professional contact; he was taking an even bigger chance by using drugs with this person while on company business.

If you're one of the millions of people who's currently unemployed, a drug arrest could affect your future employment. Think how hard it is for many people these days to land a job, given all the competition out there. Having to list a drug arrest on your job application—or to learn that it came up on a background check—is not going to help you get hired. It's going to give the other dozens, or hundreds, of other applicants an advantage over you.

So those are the potential employment costs of almost addiction. But drug use can affect you financially in many other ways. Before we wrap up this discussion on the financial costs of substance use, let's look at some figures just about the costs of nonmedical use of prescription opioids. The nonmedical use of prescription drugs is becoming a widespread problem in the United States. Nationwide, the economic costs of the nonmedical use of prescription opioids such as Vicodin, Percocet, and OxyContin totaled more than $53 billion in 2006. Of this total, $42 billion (79 percent) was due to lost productivity, $8.2 billion (15 percent) to criminal justice costs, and $2.2 billion (4 percent) to drug treatment. Another $944 million was attributable to health complications.[16]

Again, considering that drug use exists along a spectrum, some portion of these economic costs comes from people who do not carry diagnoses of either substance abuse or dependence, but who are instead almost addicted.

If you have an accident while you're high and land in the emergency room with an injury, you could be left with hundreds or thousands of dollars in medical bills that you might have avoided if you hadn't been under the influence. And again, the fact that you're not addicted won't make the bills any smaller.

The Toll on Loved Ones

If you have an almost addiction, you're probably not the only one suffering harm from it. The drug use could be affecting your spouse, parents, kids, and other loved ones, too. In one study, just under 20 percent of adults reported that drugs had caused problems within their family.[17]

In another study, from 2011, researchers found that the loved ones and significant others of substance abusers had various concerns related to the drug use. At least two-thirds of the spouses, significant others, or close family members of people who were using substances reported at least one harmful consequence. The kinds of problems caused by a family member's substance use ran the gamut of emotional, financial, health, and relationship implications.[18] Specifically, the family members cited events and issues that included

- feeling angry about the drug-using individual
- either lending money to or hiding money from the user
- being physically threatened
- finding drugs or drug paraphernalia around the house

Problems tended to be greater for women and partners of the substance user or those who were living with the substance user. What this study confirms is that the problems caused by drug use—including drug use among the almost addicted—extend beyond the users themselves and into their close relationships. The researchers didn't specifically look for families of *addicts*—they were talking to people whose loved ones had any type of substance use.

Let's return to Mike's story again. His pot smoking was a constant source of tension in his marriage. His wife Janine did not smoke marijuana and did not like that he did. She was afraid her house would be raided by the police, an understandable worry given that marijuana is illegal. She also worried that if Mike were ever caught with marijuana or arrested that it might jeopardize his career or put him in the media spotlight. Furthermore, she also worried about the impression the drug use could someday make on their child. And finally, without even knowing about his affair, she sensed that his marijuana use was yet another way in which he'd pulled away from her and their family life.

Janine's concerns highlight another observation about the relationship of substance use to marriage. At least one study has found that being married and, separately, feeling close to one's spouse may help protect against substance use. A 2009 study followed 635 people who sought help for cocaine abuse and opiate dependence. Researchers found that participants who were married used drugs on fewer days than those who weren't married. And among people who were married, those who reported having a close relationship with their spouse used less cocaine and heroin.[19]

With that study in mind, we might conclude that if Mike felt closer to his wife, he might not smoke as much marijuana or that if he didn't smoke marijuana, his wife might have a more positive impression of him.

In sum, although Mike and his family were not experiencing dramatic problems compared with some families of people who use illicit drugs, the distress that Mike's pot smoking caused Janine was real and, in the context of their marriage, definitely problematic.

If you use drugs, what might an honest look at your family and other relationships reveal about the effects of your use? For example, consider these questions:

- Do you use drugs as a way to avoid family responsibilities?
- Is your drug use a source of tension or arguments with your wife, husband, or partner?
- Has your drug use landed you in the hospital, brought the police to your door, led you to disappear for a while, or given your loved ones other reasons to worry?
- Does drug use eat into the time that you could otherwise be spending with your children?
- Could your children learn to see the appeal of illicit drugs by watching you (possibly setting the stage for addiction in your children's life)?
- Is your drug use bringing people into your life who could harm your children or cause other problems for your family?
- Could your drug use lead to a divorce or cause you to lose custody of your children? How would you feel if that happened?

Health Implications

Although the drug use of many people who are almost addicted flies well below the radar with their doctors, even nondependent drug use can have profound health implications. Consider several big-picture statistics about the health consequences of substance abuse.

In 2009, for example, people in the United States made roughly 4.6 million drug-related visits to hospital emergency departments, and almost half of those visits (45 percent) were due to drug misuse or abuse. Furthermore, in the five years leading up to 2009, ER visits involving misuse or abuse of pharmaceuticals nearly doubled, rising by 98 percent.[20]

It's not just young people who wind up on hospital tables from drug misuse. Emergency department visits by people age fifty and older that involve pharmaceutical misuse and abuse have increased rapidly. For example, between 2004 and 2008, the number of such visits increased by 121 percent to a total of 256,000 annual visits in the United States. Among the drugs that sent older people to the ER, pain relievers topped the list at 43.5 percent, followed by drugs used for anxiety or insomnia at 32 percent. More than one-third of these older patients needed to be admitted to the hospital.[21]

The health effects of illicit substance abuse are staggering, and many of these negative consequences impact the almost addicted. To begin with, a large number of adults in the United States report having driven while under the influence of an illicit substance. Data from 2006 to 2009, for instance, show that 4.3 percent of people ages sixteen or older (an estimated 10.1 million) drove under the influence of illicit drugs at some point during the previous year.[22] Impaired drivers are at high risk of life-changing traffic accidents, which can lead to hospital stays and physical rehabilitation (as well as a lengthy excursion through the legal system).

Again, if you land in a hospital ER because of an overdose, a drug that was tampered with in some way, or a bad reaction to a drug, it doesn't matter if you take drugs every day or once a week or once a month. You'll still be in the hospital, running up a big medical bill and potentially attracting attention from the authorities.

And remember, when you're buying a drug off the street, what you're buying may not actually be what the seller claims. Although there are rare stories of drugs like heroin and cocaine being "cut" (that is, diluted) with substances like rat poison, most often drugs are cut with sugars or other innocuous substances. As such, the purity of any substance can vary dramatically—including zero at times—often making it impossible to know how to "properly" dose oneself, which makes an overdose a real possibility.

I worked with one individual in his late twenties who had smoked marijuana roughly half a dozen times in his entire life. While at a party, he took a single hit of marijuana, which he later realized was probably laced with angel dust. Almost immediately upon taking the hit, he began to hallucinate, lost his balance, became disoriented, and had a horrible feeling of dread and despair. He wound up in an emergency room the next day and was given an antipsychotic medication to help relieve his symptoms. Nonetheless, his bad feelings lingered, and for several weeks he felt dread and continued to hallucinate.

This young man had mostly returned to normal within four weeks, but over the next year he would occasionally have intense flashbacks that terrified him. To my knowledge, he never smoked marijuana again.

Although this story is dramatic, it does illustrate the risks of using certain drugs even once. The upshot is that you are always taking a chance—sometimes a big one—when you ingest illicit substances.

Similarly, if you crash your vehicle while you're under the influence of a drug, the severity of your consequences won't vary depending on whether you're addicted to the drug or are just almost addicted. In that moment, all that matters is that you chose to use the drug that particular time.

I want to highlight several other facts about the health effects of illicit substance use. Many drugs of abuse—especially stimulants such as cocaine, amphetamine, and ketamine, but even marijuana for some—can cause psychotic symptoms. As such, certain people will have auditory or visual hallucinations while they are high on these drugs. Furthermore, research now clearly demonstrates that using marijuana, as well as certain other drugs of abuse, can tilt susceptible individuals toward becoming schizophrenic later in life. For example, a large 2002 study from New Zealand found that people who smoked marijuana in adolescence or young adulthood had a higher risk of developing schizophrenia or its symptoms as adults. However, this increased risk was seen mostly in those with preexisting psychotic symptoms; it was deemed nonsignificant for those with no such symptoms before using marijuana.[23]

Furthermore, the risk is dose-dependent, meaning the more marijuana you smoke, the greater your risk. For example, a study of young Swedes found that people who had already used marijuana more than fifty times increased their risk of schizophrenia by a factor of six (600 percent). Those who had used it only five to ten times increased their risk by 70 percent.[24] People could easily use marijuana ten times, or even fifty times or more, and still not meet the criteria for addiction.

More recently, a 2009 review article looked at data from seven studies. One study found no greater risk of developing psychosis after low-level marijuana use, but the other studies all found a heightened risk, especially for those already vulnerable to the illness.[25] So it appears that people who are vulnerable almost certainly have a higher risk of psychosis, while those less susceptible may also have some added risk—and either way, the risk is dose-dependent. Does this mean that marijuana users in the almost addicted range have a greater risk for psychosis? That question may be debatable, but why take the chance?

Marijuana may also increase the risk of becoming depressed or anxious later in life. One Australian study, for example, found that teens who used marijuana weekly or more frequently nearly doubled their risk for later depression or anxiety.[26] As we'll see later in this book, people may cope with depression or anxiety by turning to drugs. In addition, as many comedies on TV and film have demonstrated, marijuana use can also cause long-lasting memory deficits, though this is rarely as amusing in real life as it is on the screen.

Again, the more extensive the drug use, the more likely it is that these problems and conditions may develop. But any drug use is a potential threat from a health perspective, and no use can ever be considered completely safe. For example, sports fans may remember that in 1986, Len Bias, a University of Maryland basketball player who'd just been drafted second overall by the Boston Celtics, died of a cardiac arrhythmia after using cocaine. He apparently was otherwise the picture of health when he died and is considered by many to be one of the best basketball players ever to not play professionally.

Moreover, many illicit drugs lower people's inhibitions and increase their likelihood of engaging in risky behavior. Not surprisingly then, drug use among teenagers increases their chances of becoming pregnant and contracting HIV (human immunodeficiency virus) or other sexually transmitted diseases. Similarly, drug use places people at risk of becoming victims of violence. I've heard many stories from patients of all ages who developed illnesses and injuries related in some way to their drug use.

In Mike's case, on the night of his arrest he had smoked marijuana and consumed a fair amount of alcohol. The combination of the two drugs no doubt slowed down his reflexes, and it is possible that if he'd been clean and sober, he wouldn't have gotten into the vehicle accident. He's fortunate that neither he nor the other driver were injured beyond being shaken up, which is an outcome that could have easily occurred.

Legal Implications

Let's not forget that except for alcohol and legitimately prescribed drugs, including in some specific instances marijuana, using drugs is generally against the law. Whether you agree that drugs should be illegal or not, any use of an illicit substance is inherently risky from a legal perspective.

I have known professionals with high-profile jobs who lost their ability to work in their profession because they were found with illicit drugs. Although some might deem marijuana to be especially benign, that doesn't mean that physicians who are caught possessing it a single time won't be charged with a crime, possibly removed from their positions temporarily or permanently, and likely forced into a treatment program followed by a monitoring program to ensure abstinence for several years—even if they were infrequent users. For lawyers, being convicted of possessing an illicit substance could result in the revocation of their bar membership, thereby jeopardizing their ability to practice law and provide for themselves and their families.

Almost addiction can also expose someone to the legal system via the relationship between drug use and other crimes. Federal government statistics show that adults arrested for a serious offense in the past year were more likely to have used an illicit drug that year than people who weren't arrested (60.1 versus 13.6 percent).[27]

A 2009 survey on drug use among men who had been arrested in ten metropolitan areas across the United States found that as many as 87 percent of arrestees tested positive for an illicit drug—a figure far higher than statistics for the general population. The most common substances found during tests, in descending order, were marijuana, cocaine, opiates, and methamphetamine. In addition, many arrestees had been using more than one substance—with figures ranging from 15 percent in Atlanta to 40 percent in Chicago.[28]

How many of these users were addicted and how many were almost addicted? Again, it doesn't really matter; what does matter is that they all put drugs into their body. And that's something that's true for both people who are almost addicted and people with true addictions. Though the typical person who's almost addicted isn't robbing convenience stores to pay for a drug habit, otherwise stable and reasonable people may behave in an unreasonable manner when under the influence, which could set the stage for mischief and violence.

Like many middle- and upper-class marijuana smokers, Mike said he never worried much about the fact that marijuana is illegal. He'd had a steady supplier for years whom he trusted, so he didn't have to venture into sketchy situations to obtain it. And he knew how to be discreet about his marijuana use. Despite all these supposed safeguards, all it would take was a disgruntled mistress—or an angry wife contemplating divorce— to alert the authorities and turn Mike's marijuana use into a noose with which to hang him.

Almost Addicted No More: Steps to Take Now

Perhaps you suspect that you are almost addicted but are still weighing the evidence one way or the other. If you're a friend or loved one of someone who is almost addicted, you may be building a case for confronting this person. In either situation, a good place to start is by considering whether the drug use has already led to the type of problems we've discussed in this chapter.

Find Out How Drugs Have Impacted Your Life

First, if you use drugs, examine the ways that even casual use may have impacted your life. Go through the following questions with care, and be honest. If you can't answer any of the questions with certainty, consider asking a friend or family member to help. (And make note of any points where you agree that drug use has caused a problem. Having this information on hand will be useful later if you're reminding yourself why you need to quit.)

Work or School Repercussions
Have you ever

- given less than your full effort at work or school because you used drugs?
- written work emails that you later regretted while you were under the influence of drugs?

- been reprimanded at work for performance issues?
- been asked at work if you got enough sleep?
- signed a deal while under the influence?
- divulged a business secret while under the influence?
- berated your boss or co-workers in a way you'd never do if you were clean and sober?
- submitted shoddy work or schoolwork because of drug use?
- been called to the dean's office because of something that occurred while you were using drugs or alcohol?

Family Repercussions
Have you ever
- deliberately broken something of value around the home?
- been asked by your family to stop using drugs?
- been told by your family that you were acting strangely?
- embarrassed your family due to drugs?
- missed an important family function due to drug use?
- used drugs in front of your child or been under the influence around your child?
- yelled at or berated a family member while under the influence, only to regret it once sober?
- cheated on a partner or spouse with someone while you were under the influence and regretted it later? (I should note here that I never felt that Mike was having his affair with Ana *because* of his substance use. Instead, the substance use merely added layers of complexity onto the affair and potential threat to Mike's work and family life.)

Legal Repercussions

Have you ever

- been arrested for drug use or possession?
- worried about being arrested because of your drug use?
- had to hastily hide or discard drugs because law enforcement was approaching?
- committed a crime in order to pay for your drug use, even if you weren't caught?

Health Repercussions

Have you ever

- injured yourself while high?
- skipped a planned workout because of drugs?
- forgotten to take a prescribed medication because of your substance use?
- downplayed—or lied about—your substance use to a health care provider for fear of consequences of various sorts, including getting a lecture?
- went to an emergency room because of something that happened while you were using drugs?
- caught a sexually transmitted disease because of sex you had while under the influence?
- had sex that you later regretted while on drugs?

If you (or a loved one) are almost addicted, your answers to these questions may be enough to convince you that a change is necessary. If you're reading this for yourself, why might you want to alter your behavior and change your relationship to drugs? The most basic reason is that deep down, you know that something is wrong. Your drug use is still manageable, but you feel that an unlucky incident could knock your life off the rails. Maybe your drug use has caused problems for you one too many times.

What can you do to make that leap and admit that your drug use, even though it doesn't rise to the level of substance abuse or addiction, is troublesome and therefore needs to change? As hard as it might be, acknowledging the extent of problems that your drug use has caused is a good first step. *Maybe drugs* did *cause me to blow off my son's Little League game. Maybe my husband was right when he said that drugs are keeping me from caring for my family properly. Maybe drugs are the reason my career just hasn't taken off.* These kinds of realizations have started plenty of people down the path to cleaning drugs out of their lives.

We know that if you've become accustomed to taking drugs, you're probably conflicted about even looking at the issue, much less making any changes. But ask yourself as honestly as possible: Have any problems resulted from my drug use? Are there any gaps or discrepancies between my current behaviors and the goals I've set for myself?

It is understandable and actually expected that you feel resistance to even answering these questions. After all, who stands up and volunteers, "I have a major problem that needs addressing"? It is natural to resist this kind of questioning and dialogue and to downplay the negative consequences of your drug use. If need be, start by asking yourself just one question: Do I have any possible reason, even just one, to change?

Where You Are and Where You Want to Be

Take a look at where you are in your life. Consider your accomplishments: Are you satisfied with where you are in your work and personal life? Think about how you spend your time: Are you getting through life in an organized manner and meeting your obligations? Think about your emotional state: Is depression or anxiety interfering with your happiness or productivity? Could any old hurts or traumas be influencing your decisions?

If you sense that your life could be better in some way, try to determine specifically what you would like to see improved. Would you like to spend more time reading with your kids? Would you like to tend to your obligations with less rush? Would you like to live in the moment more, rather than replaying the past or dreading the future? Come up with specific, measurable goals for where you'd like your life to be: for example, "I'd like to make all of my kids' softball games this summer, and I would like to bounce out of bed with energy each morning."

Now, consider whether your drug use will interfere with meeting those goals—even to a small degree. Ask yourself if your drug use is slowing you down, taking up valuable time, or masking the roots of your anxiety or depression. If so, that's a pretty good endorsement that you need to ditch the drugs to meet your goals.

Mike's Outcome

Well, let me make known up front that psychiatrists, including myself, do not bat 1,000—we do not always succeed. Although Mike benefited from having a sounding board about his marriage and his affair, he never came to see anything wrong with his marijuana use except that it caused friction between him and his wife. In our sessions over eight months, I couldn't find a foothold regarding his marijuana use that would lead him to conclude he needed to quit smoking it.

Mike got lucky that his brush with the law due to his substance use didn't cause long-term damage to his life. Things also worked out when he decided that he needed to focus on his marriage and leave Ana. Though she was unhappy, she never divulged Mike's drug use—or his other secrets—to his employer.

But as long as marijuana is a part of his life, leaving him vulnerable to arrest or for his employers to question his judgment, Mike's almost addiction could certainly lead to his downfall in the future.

■ ◆ ■

Part 2

The Roots of Almost Addiction

3

Almost Addiction
When the Past Influences the Present

A jumble of influences and factors can lead people to become almost addicted, including boredom, excitement, a desire to fit in with others, and a family history of substance use. In this chapter, I'll look into some of these root causes. This can help you identify what may have influenced your almost addiction or that of a loved one and give you clues on how to create solutions. In addition, this chapter will take a look at how drugs affect the brain, which will allow you to better understand why they can be so hard to quit.

For more insight into these issues, I'll begin with the story of a patient I'll call Alexa.

Alexa's Story

Alexa had graduated from medical school a few years earlier and was finishing her residency training in internal medicine when she came to see me. The most immediate reason that she had landed in my office was that she was engaged to a man, Harold, who had several children from his first marriage. Although she loved Harold, she found herself confused, conflicted, jealous, and at times angry about his healthy relationship with his children, especially his daughters. The adult part of her knew that most of her feelings were irrational, but they'd taken such a hold on her that she was distraught at a time when she should have been happy and excited.

Beneath Alexa's confused, troubled feelings lay a lot of history and baggage. Raised in a small midwestern town, she had never met her father. When her mother was seven months pregnant, he left her for a younger woman. When I met her, Alexa didn't even know if her father was alive or dead.

Alexa's mother had been sexually abused by an uncle during her childhood and teenage years. After high school, she married her boyfriend but the relationship ended in divorce. She later married Alexa's father. After Alexa's birth, her mother likely developed postpartum depression, and she wasn't able to care for Alexa. She soon attempted suicide and thereafter spent time in a psychiatric unit. Between the ages of two and eight, Alexa was moved from one relative's house to another.

During this time, the family history repeated itself. Alexa was repeatedly sexually molested by an older male cousin, who had alcohol abuse problems, as she later learned. She also experienced several more instances of abuse involving other people.

At age eight, Alexa moved in with her mother and new stepfather. Unlike many of the men in her life until this point, the stepfather was kind toward her and did what he could to protect and nurture Alexa. Her mother, always bitter and stern, insisted that Alexa would go to college, then medical school, and return to their small midwestern town to serve as a family doctor for the community. Alexa described her mother as "impossible to please," but she would also readily defend her because of the traumatic upbringing she'd had.

In high school, Alexa took advanced courses and made straight As. But while she was achieving academically, other parts of her life were faltering. Near the end of her sophomore year, she became anorexic and, within a year, developed bulimia, leading her to binge and purge at least once a day. The bulimia continued until the end of medical school.

In her sophomore year of college, she began dating a senior, Ben, who she thought exuded an aura of coolness and adventure. Like Alexa, Ben and his friends were excellent students who were destined for graduate and professional schools. Yet, Ben also made time for drugs and alcohol, which he introduced to Alexa. She tried nearly everything—though she never used opiate painkillers and avoided injecting—and found that while she didn't particularly like alcohol or marijuana, she did find hallucinogens and some stimulants (especially cocaine) very appealing. During her last two years of college, Alexa used drugs every week or two.

Despite having several options closer to her home, after college she moved East for medical school. She wasn't consciously aware of it at the time, but moving away from the Midwest was probably her first effort to break free of her mother's tight grip. During her first year of medical school, Alexa excelled academically but continued to binge and purge, and she still used various drugs occasionally.

Near the end of her first year, and throughout her second year of medical school, Alexa's drug of choice became cocaine and she used it exclusively. At her peak, she was snorting it weekly. She noticed that it made her feel good, enabled her to study late into the night, and helped her cope with the stress of medical school. She would later acknowledge that when she was coming off cocaine, the lethargy from the crash was often hard to shake.

Around this time, Alexa began to question her relationship with her mother. As with anyone who undergoes a conversion, the change began with various small observations and then progressed to bigger, potentially life-altering questions: Why didn't her mother ever seem happy? Why wasn't her mother ever pleased with her accomplishments? Did Alexa really want to be a doctor at all, or was she in medical school because of her mother's pressure?

During a phone conversation with her mother after her first year of medical school, she began asking some of these questions. Instead of taking her concerns seriously, her mother instead asked Alexa who had put these ideas into her head.

Along with questioning this relationship, Alexa began seeing the problems that cocaine was causing. She began to realize that the drug—which she never took before class or before working in the clinic—made her feel good in the moment but also was dragging her down. She'd be exhausted the day after doing coke and sometimes had trouble concentrating.

Knowing that her life was heading off track, she went to see a counselor, who quickly targeted Alexa's relationship with her mother as the central culprit in her eating disorders. (Even though she was a bright doctor-to-be, like many people with anorexia or bulimia, Alexa initially thought she was the only person who'd ever starved herself or thrown up on purpose.)

Around this time, Alexa finally came to see cocaine as something she could never use again, because it was just too appealing for her. She was driving back from a solo camping weekend in the mountains. It was dusk and she had snorted a line of cocaine just before getting in the car to leave. She had left the remainder in a baggie on the backseat next to a duffel bag with her clothing and some textbooks. Close to home, a police car pulled up behind her and flashed its lights. As she was pulling over, panic set in—her chest began pounding, her head spinning—as she realized that the cocaine was still in her system and moreover was visible in her car. She thought her medical career was about to end before it even got started. The officer pulled in behind her, opened his door, and strode toward her car. She took several deep breaths and rolled down her window, fearing the worst.

Nonchalantly, the officer told her that one of her taillights wasn't working and that she should get it fixed immediately. With little fanfare, he issued her a written warning and departed.

Alexa never did cocaine again. During that police stop, she realized that coke was too dangerous to even think about using—her entire career could be shot down if she were caught.

She freely told me that although she had almost completely stopped taking illicit drugs by the time she came to see me, hallucinogens still appealed to her because she felt that they made her more aware of herself in relation to her mother, as well as raising her consciousness in general. She said she still used them if she came across them but, living in a new city and not being one to go out of her way to procure them, she didn't have any easy access to these drugs. Regardless, she told me that cocaine was far too dangerous to ever use again because it appealed to her just a little too much.

The Role of Family History in Substance Use

For many people, their family history can reliably create a map of their future. Because of this, my advice to virtually everyone is that they ought to choose their parents well. They should choose their grandparents well, too, although that's a bit tougher.

Kidding aside, I can't stress enough how much your biological family history plays a role in your chance of developing problems with drugs. A predilection for substance problems runs in families. People with relatives who are substance-dependent are much more likely to become addicted themselves (or almost addicted), even if they are raised apart from the family members who abuse drugs.

How does this happen? Several mechanisms play a role in how families influence one's drug use. Although it might sound strange, perhaps the most fundamental way that this tendency gets passed along is directly through the genes.

Researchers have repeatedly shown that genes can predispose people toward problematic substance use. Studies of twins, for example, have revealed that children of parents who are addicted are much more likely than others to develop addictive disorders themselves, even if they are adopted into families that do not have any problems with substances. In fact, genetic factors may be responsible for 30 to 60 percent of the overall difference in risk of drug addiction between people.[29]

In addition to a direct risk of developing addiction, your genes may also influence how likely you are to engage in risky or impulsive behaviors, which indirectly increases your chances of problematic substance use. Your genes also influence the way you respond to stressful events, so that some people are more prone to becoming anxious or fearful in certain circumstances than others, another trait that might lead to drug use. And your genes play a role in your chance of developing depression, which, like anxiety, is found in many people with addictions or almost addiction (the next chapter will discuss how people with almost addiction often use drugs as an unhealthy coping mechanism for depression, anxiety, and other mental issues.)[30]

In Alexa's case, several family members—including the uncle who abused her mother and the cousin who molested her—had problems with substance use. Although alcohol was the drug of choice in both of these cases, there is reason to think that any form of addiction in a family increases the risk of other addictions among that group.

The environment of a family can also "pass down" drug use from generation to generation. When a child grows up watching family members use drugs, the child may develop a skewed concept of what normal drug-related behaviors look like. It's like the 1980s TV commercial in which a father confronts his teenage son about the boy's drug stash, asking "Where did you learn how to use drugs?" The boy responds, "I learned it by watching *you!*"

I have had dozens of patients—many of them raised by parents who smoke marijuana—tell me in all seriousness that "everyone" smokes pot. They don't mean everyone they know. They mean *everyone*, period.

When I ask for clarification (and I always do), they will repeat that phrase to me and tell me they don't know a single person who doesn't smoke pot. Furthermore, children who grow up watching their loved ones smoke, inject, or swallow illicit drugs might not even know until they are older that these drugs are against the law and that, therefore, any use whatsoever is potentially problematic.

There are other ways that a childhood spent in the presence of drug use might lead kids to develop warped views of events. To them, seeing someone intoxicated or otherwise checked out from reality is the norm rather than the exception.

Consider a scenario in which a wife is in denial about her husband's substance use and when her son sees Dad passed out on the front lawn and begs Mother to help, instead of calling 911 or thanking the child for his concern, the mother informs her son that Dad isn't passed out but is, in fact, just napping. After several episodes like this, the child begins to learn that he cannot trust his senses and cannot be sure about the accuracy of his perceptions.

As a result, kids who grew up in such environments might have warped perceptions about people's relationship with substances and think that certain behaviors are normal instead of significantly outside customary behavior. They might not even be aware that they have this view, but they may have an underlying sense that "drug use is okay, and it doesn't really cause problems," which influences their behaviors.

Beyond the genetic influences that one inherits, or the ways that family members model drug use to a child, families can influence substance use in still other ways.

Specifically, if a parent chronically abuses drugs and as a result is not fully present to support the family and help solve its problems, children might experience neglect, be vulnerable to abuse, or simply form a very poor attachment to the parent. And these experiences can actually permanently change the way these kids' brains work.

It makes sense: parents' basic job is to protect and nurture their children and provide a safe, loving environment from which they can explore the world. So if children feel abandoned, neglected, and alone because of poor parenting, it's not hard to guess why they would turn to a substance—or a bad relationship or some other troubling behavior—to create an artificial sense of warmth and belonging, given that a real one just isn't there.

Science supports this observation. One study, for example, found that ninth graders who were unsupervised after school were more likely to smoke tobacco and marijuana and were also more likely to drink alcohol. Kids who were poorly supervised at home were more likely to engage in risky behaviors. Conversely, children whose parents were more engaged in their lives exhibited fewer risky behaviors and less substance use.[31]

Weak parenting seems to be a factor in Alexa's drug use. She certainly suffered from neglect—her father disappeared before she was even born, and her mother left her in the "care" of various relatives.

Under these living conditions, Alexa was exposed to repeated sexual abuse and trauma at the hands of family and strangers. Given that she lacked a sustained loving and nurturing parental presence, as well as experienced overt abuse, it's not surprising that Alexa became almost addicted to cocaine and possibly other drugs.

The Initial Appeal of Drugs

The reasons people use drugs are probably as varied as the people who use them. That said, over and over in my practice, I have seen clients engaged in drug use who were self-medicating their depression, anxiety, or other mood, emotional, or focus disorders. I've known plenty of individuals who were predisposed toward depression—you might say they have depressive personalities—whose use of drugs momentarily lifted them out of the prison of their low mood.

In the same manner, when someone is prone to anxiety, many substances of abuse calm them (especially drugs that slow the mind like benzodiazepines, alcohol, or marijuana). I have also seen some people with psychotic processes, such as hearing voices in their heads or seeing things that weren't really there, who viewed illicit drugs as a salve for their psychiatric troubles. Again, we'll cover these common reasons for drug use in more detail in the next chapter.

It is also possible that those who are more likely to use drugs and find them especially appealing are more prone to feeling awkward, angry, or impatient than others. For individuals with these characteristics, using drugs may help normalize their appearance and mood.

People who enjoy using illicit drugs might also be more impulsive than others. Impulsive individuals either don't or can't comprehend the potential consequences of risky behaviors; as a result, they view the immediate excitement surrounding drugs as far more compelling than the threat of jail time, a tapped-out bank account, poor credit, a communicable disease, or an unplanned pregnancy.

Another trait common to many people who are almost

addicted is a need for excitement or thrills. Timid individuals—those who are careful to protect themselves physically and emotionally—are much less likely to engage in high-risk behavior designed to produce an immediate thrill; as such, they have a lower risk of initial drug use.

Similarly, although you can find plenty of exceptions, many people who use illicit drugs enjoy nonconformity and look down on behaviors considered "normal." This value, along with a feeling of alienation from mainstream culture, can produce attitudes that disparage "straight" people and their lifestyles as boring.

Alexa started using drugs for various reasons, including some of the factors just discussed. The conflict she experienced with her mother and the abuse from her childhood probably set her up for some degree of depression and anxiety, even if it was underlying her stable exterior. She obviously felt pain on some level, evident in her long-term eating-disordered behaviors. Certainly her boyfriend and his friends prided themselves on being nonconformist, and their drug use was one way of standing out from the crowd.

Alexa had a lifetime of challenges that were weighing on her mind, even if some of the burden was affecting her on a deep level she could barely recognize. But emerging scientific research suggests that Alexa's brain—the physical organ—was responding to drugs in a way that encouraged her to continue using. Her dopamine system was likely out of balance, leaving her more vulnerable to the soothing and pleasurable effects of drugs.

To understand almost addiction requires an appreciation of the brain chemical dopamine. Let's take a closer look.

Dopamine, Drugs, and the Brain during Almost Addiction

Dopamine is a neurotransmitter in the central nervous system (that is, the brain) that carries messages from one nerve cell to another. Dopamine also serves as a stimulant. This means that if you shower a brain with dopamine, in general, the owner of that brain is going to feel good. Inject dopamine into an intravenous line heading into someone's vein, and her heart rate is going to increase and her blood pressure is going to rise. Not surprisingly then, dopamine in excess is harmful. If too much hits your heart, it can overstress the organ and you could have a heart attack and die. Too much in the brain can overstimulate it too. You can become acutely psychotic, paranoid, or overwhelmingly anxious from too much dopamine, which is almost always followed by a hard crash that results in fatigue, drowsiness, and depression.

Almost all drugs of abuse stimulate what is called a *reward pathway* in the brain by increasing the activity of dopamine. Other pleasurable activities also activate and excite this reward pathway, like eating an excellent meal or having sex. Many elements influence the degree to which you're able to be excited by dopaminergic (the medical term for dopamine-related) activity, such as genetic, environmental, cognitive, and emotional factors.

Remember that people's genes and environment affect both their likelihood of developing problems with their ways of thinking and problems with drugs. In Alexa's case, for example, substance use ran in her family, as did psychiatric disorders. Alexa's mother almost certainly had post-traumatic stress disorder and her grandmother, as I learned from our talks, likely suffered from depression.

Any behavior exhibited or experienced in the external world has direct, real physiological effects in the brain. In other words, events in your surroundings can make lasting changes in your brain itself. So it is not surprising that the dopamine system in someone who has experienced trauma or abuse can be dysfunctional. The dysregulated dopamine system in these individuals could then predispose them to developing substance use disorders.[32]

Research has shown that childhood neglect and physical or sexual victimization are associated with later adolescent alcohol, marijuana, and inhalant use.[33] Thus, the interaction between difficult, painful, and abusive circumstances and subsequent drug use disorders appears evident—and dopamine could play a role in the connection.

Drugs, Dopamine, and Danger

Your brain needs a certain level of dopamine, but too much interferes with its proper function. In vulnerable people, excessive dopamine can cause anxiety or agitation, mania, and even psychosis.

Amphetamine drugs trigger the release of massive amounts of dopamine, along with another excitatory neurotransmitter that your body makes from dopamine called norepinephrine. This is a close cousin of epinephrine—also called adrenaline—and like dopamine, it switches all your systems to "on." Your heart rate increases, oxygen levels in your brain go up, and your blood glucose (blood sugar) levels rise. The end effect is that your body is revved up and ready to rumble.

When most people use a drug like cocaine or amphetamine, they are hoping to feel euphoria. But if you get even a tad too much—and for some folks "too much" might be "any at all"—

you can cross over into the downsides of these drugs, which include insomnia, irritability, weakness, dizziness, and tremors. As if that's not enough, such drugs can also cause confusion, delirium, panic, and suicidal tendencies, especially in people who are mentally ill.[34]

Since the brains of people who regularly use amphetamine or other stimulating drugs are overexcited from the flood of dopamine, their brains do what they can to maintain equilibrium. One way they do this is to decrease the number of dopamine uptake sites in the brain—the places on neurons (nerve cells) that allow dopamine to take action. A lower number of these sites means dopamine has fewer areas where it can affect the brain.

Another way brains protect themselves is by lowering the levels of a dopamine building block called tyrosine hydroxylase, which means that the ingredients needed to make dopamine are less available. Fewer ingredients, then, mean less dopamine will be produced. This "down regulation" explains why users may require ever-increasing amounts of a drug to get the same high.

The crash that people feel when coming down from cocaine or crystal meth or other amphetamines is related to dopamine as well, but in this case, a lack of the stuff. Dopamine stores become depleted because much of the body's supply of dopamine is released during the excitation and stimulation from these drugs. Afterward, the system cannot produce enough dopamine to replace the used-up brain chemical. So not only are the body's stores of dopamine depleted, but the ingredients needed to make more are lacking. Plus, the tiny "doorways" in the brain's cells that allow dopamine to enter and take action—the receptor sites—are diminished. The result is the lethargy, depression, and sexual dysfunction that is often seen during amphetamine or other stimulant withdrawal.

These effects have been demonstrated in animal experiments. Research has found that amphetamine not only caused dopamine depletion in certain areas of mice's brains, but it also led to brain cell death in these areas.[35] Dopamine itself also appears to be *neurotoxic*—or harmful to neurons in excessive amounts—so that after a large continuous release of dopamine, neurons do not function normally and become somewhat accustomed to the effects of dopamine. As a result, the brain might need a larger amount of dopamine just to feel normal.

Why is all of this business about dopamine so important when we're talking about almost addiction? Because it's essential to remember that illicit drug use doesn't just affect the mental functioning of people with hard-core addiction. Even if you use drugs only occasionally, your use is still affecting the way your brain works at a very fundamental level.

Not only that, you are changing the way your brain works by exposing it to chemicals that may be unregulated, impure, stronger than you were expecting, and not taken under the supervision of someone with training in pharmacology or medicine (you know, the kind of person you'd want messing with your brain chemicals).

You may have a lot on your mind from past traumas or adversities that have been passed down in your family. Nonetheless, revving your brain up and letting it crash down, over and over, with the use of illicit drugs is just causing you more harm—and leaving you less able to cope with your problems in a healthy manner.

Drug-Free Strategies for Coping
with Difficulties in Your Life

We've talked in this chapter about some of the factors that may influence people to use drugs, as you saw with Alexa, who turned to cocaine and hallucinogens. These include family history of drug use and past trauma.

Now it's time to take a hard look at yourself and consider whether these are issues in your life. For starters, does drug abuse or dependence run in your family? Although earlier I advised you to choose your parents wisely if you want to avoid family-related health issues, you can't really do this. Even if you really wish that your ancestry had been otherwise, unfortunately you can't go back and apply for a new set of parents or transplant someone else's DNA into your body.

So what can you do to help yourself if you realize that your family tree is loaded with substance abuse issues?

You can be vigilant.

People learn all the time that their family history has put them at higher risk of chronic conditions, such as heart disease. In addition, other factors may increase people's risk of heart problems—things they can't do a single thing about, like their age and race. For people in these situations, it's important to change the many, many risk factors that they *can* do something about, like their weight, diet, exercise habits, blood pressure, cholesterol, and whether they drink excessively or smoke.

The same is true for people whose family background increases their risk of becoming almost addicted. If this is your story, it's in your best interest to be extra cautious around drugs to avoid stepping over any line and becoming almost addicted or worse. In fact, for anyone with a family history of substance use problems, displaying an abundance of caution about drugs should be the rule. If the average person is wary about using drugs, you should steer away from drugs and situations where people are using them with an added degree of caution. If you suspect that illicit drugs represent a shiny lure that could hook you like a fish, you should consider a consultation with a mental health provider soon after you begin using them.

If you've been physically, sexually, or emotionally abused at any point in your life, and your drug use has reached the almost addicted stage, it's a good idea to seek outside help for those old traumas as well. That goes for abuse that involved family members, friends, or strangers, and abuse that occurred in childhood or adulthood. It's very possible that you may be using drugs—or the situations or people you encounter while using or obtaining drugs—to respond to those hurts.

Finding help for emotional trauma might provide, as a starting point, the realization that you are not alone. Trauma is often very isolating by its nature, but knowing that others also have experienced trauma, and that the loved ones around you care about you, is all-important. Asking anyone in your circle—friends, family, or clergy—for support can be lifesaving. Support groups, online and in person, specifically for survivors of abuse may also be helpful. The people you'll meet along these paths will likely remind you that using drugs is not a healthy way to cope with hurtful factors in your life.

Attending to your basic health needs is also vital, because if your physical health fails, you're apt to run into emotional trouble. As such, eating right, getting adequate sleep, exercising, and regularly visiting your primary care doctor are all vital.

I'll touch on all of those in the next chapter, which addresses the link between almost addiction and depression and anxiety.

Alexa's Outcome

It's worth remembering that Alexa did not come to see me because she was worried about her past or present drug use. Rather, she sought out a psychiatrist because of her feelings about her fiancé's relationship with his children, and so we initially focused on that.

Although she was not a teetotaler or someone who swore off all drug use, by the time I met her, she had already determined that the lure of cocaine for her was so strong that she could never use it again. I agreed: at the height of her use, she had been almost addicted to cocaine.

I didn't need to possess the clinical insight of Sigmund Freud to realize fairly quickly that Alexa's reaction to her fiancé's relationship with his kids confused and troubled her in various ways. She had never known her father, and her new life with her fiancé and his children repeatedly hammered home that fact for her. Not only that, but her fiancé loved, supported, and protected his daughters, which further dredged up a confusing swirl of emotions within her, given that she had been harmed in her life by an older male relative.

Alexa felt jealous of the girls, because she thought her fiancé couldn't possibly have enough love to go around. "If he loves them," Alexa said of the kids, "how can he love me too?"

Alexa and I met roughly two dozen times over the course of a year—her residency schedule limited the time she had to meet—and we met jointly with her fiancé once as well. At this session, he reassured her that he did indeed love his kids and wanted to remain very present in their lives, but that he also deeply adored Alexa.

Over time, Alexa came to trust that Harold had enough love to go around for everyone. When we last met, the young doctor had not forced herself to vomit, as part of her eating disorder, in six months. She also abstained from cocaine throughout the time I knew her. She did drink alcohol on occasion and once took hallucinatory mushrooms during the year we worked together, but she never suffered from any substance-related problems.

Although she had spent part of her life in almost addiction, which could have destroyed her medical career before it even started, she was able to successfully move away from it.

❖

4

Double Trouble

Almost Addiction and Mental Health Issues

If you drew a circle representing people who have mental health issues and another circle representing those who use illicit drugs, the circles would have a substantial overlap. Many people who seek treatment for a psychiatric issue also take illicit substances, and conversely, many who seek treatment for some kind of substance use disorder also have some type of psychiatric issue.

For lack of another umbrella term that sounds less clinical than "psychiatric disorder," the rest of this chapter will generally refer to such problems, including depression, anxiety, and attention deficit hyperactivity disorder (ADHD), as "mental health issues."

When individuals have both a mental health issue and a substance problem, their chances of being successfully treated for either diminishes considerably. This means that people working to conquer almost addiction should be well aware of the possibility that they have a coexisting mental health issue. And, if so, they should be ready to confront it head-on.

Despite this large overlap, or perhaps because of it, a separate mental health issue is very easy to miss in someone who is using drugs. When a person is directly under the influence of a drug or is coming off one, the symptoms of intoxication or withdrawal can resemble many cognitive or mood problems, including depression, anxiety, mania, disorientation, confusion, or even psychosis. To further complicate matters, drug use itself can actually cause a full-blown psychiatric disorder to develop. Because of these various possibilities, when someone who is using or abusing drugs and also exhibiting psychiatric symptoms meets with a mental health care provider for the first time, that professional can have a difficult time teasing apart which problem came first and whether one might have caused the other. So as you're investigating any factors involved in your almost addiction—or a loved one's almost addiction—it's crucial to acknowledge and investigate any mood, attention, or other mental health issues that may be playing a role.

For a case in point, I'd like to share the story of Evan, a young man in his twenties who came into my clinic, mostly against his will.

Evan's Story

Evan was on leave from college, and his parents, who supported him financially, told him that if he didn't undergo drug testing and enter treatment for substance abuse, they'd cut him off. So he sat in my office but wasn't willing to do much more, such as talk openly.

At our first meeting, no matter how I posed questions about his drug use, Evan would do everything he could to avoid providing any useful information. In subsequent visits he did begin to talk, but although we eventually established some rapport, he always downplayed his drug use—whatever he did admit to taking was probably less than what he was actually using.

Both of Evan's parents were professionals who'd risen from modest beginnings to a comfortable life in an affluent suburb of Boston. His father was a partner in a major architectural firm, and his mother was a former public school teacher who had become a principal at one of the better Boston-area public schools.

When I first met Evan, he told me that he used "basically nothing" and that his parents were unnecessarily up in arms about his drug use. Whenever a patient says something to the effect that his drug use amounts to "*almost* nothing" or "*basically* zero," the only thing I conclude with certainty is that the person is using drugs rather than *not* using drugs.

I've seen patients whose "almost nothing" was in fact almost nothing and others for whom "practically zero" actually meant daily drug use. As a clinical matter, when a patient tells me, usually at an initial meeting, that he drinks a six-pack a day, I will respond with a somewhat distracted-appearing, low-key response like, "You mean a case of beer a day?" preferably with my eyes averted. (A case contains twenty-four beers.) Occasionally I'll get a response like, "No, I mean a six-pack," but more often I will hear something like, "Not a case. I almost never drink more than eighteen beers a day."

Only rarely do patients seem offended by my principle of quadrupling whatever they self-report as their drug intake.

(Parents and other concerned family members may want to keep this approach in mind when they discuss almost addiction with a loved one!)

So given that Evan's parents were "freaking out" and that he used some drugs rather than none, I had to keep hunting. He admitted that he first used marijuana at age sixteen and after that only smoked pot irregularly. He said that never in his life had he smoked on a daily basis, and he couldn't remember doing it as much as three times in a single week.

Evan gave the impression that he currently used marijuana maybe once every two weeks, but that he had essentially quit since his parents insisted on starting drug testing a couple of months earlier. He also told me that he very rarely drank and that he'd never had a problem with alcohol. Since starting drug testing, he said he'd stopped drinking entirely. He also told me that he had never used any other drugs, including opiates, cocaine, hallucinogens, or inhalants.

The story his parents told, however, included some convincing circumstantial evidence that this young man might be crushing and snorting stimulants. When they had dropped by his apartment for an unannounced visit several months earlier, they'd discovered a pill crusher, several straws, and rolled-up tubes of paper. More than once they'd observed him examining his face very closely in a mirror, which they later concluded was him looking for powder residue. Despite his parents' observations, Evan maintained his denial that he'd never used anything other than marijuana or alcohol.

Although the facts of Evan's drug use remained murky, his psychiatric history was much less so. Veins of significant illness ran throughout both sides of his family. Several relatives on his mother's side had both anxiety and panic disorder, and his father's side of the family was rife with depression, with at least one family member having bipolar disorder. In addition, Evan had several relatives who heavily abused substances.

As you learned from Alexa's story in the last chapter, knowing a person's family history is very important for a doctor when considering substance abuse or psychiatric illness. The likelihood of developing a problem in either arena increases—sometimes dramatically—when a person has relatives with a given condition.

As Evan told his story, he touched on seeing a psychiatrist starting at age ten, getting a diagnosis of ADHD—or maybe dyslexia, he said—and starting a prescription of stimulant medication. Since that time, he'd been on one stimulant or another nearly continuously. During his teen years he was also diagnosed with depression and anxiety, and he had been put on a number of medications for those conditions as well. He couldn't remember all of the prescriptions his doctors had tried, but his list included an array of familiar names: Strattera, Ritalin, Zoloft, Wellbutrin, Celexa, Lexapro, Ativan, Adderall, and Seroquel.

He also downplayed the extent of his depression and anxiety, yet his symptoms were serious enough at age seventeen that he was hospitalized for depression for a week. His classroom attendance in both high school and college was spotty, and he'd had trouble showing up for work consistently since going on leave from college.

When I first met with Evan, he stared straight ahead throughout much of our visit, making inconsistent eye contact. He also showed little facial expression or emotion throughout the meeting.

I diagnosed him with ADHD by history (since there was no evidence of symptoms during my meeting with him), depressive disorder, anxiety disorder, and possible Asperger's syndrome (sort of a mild form of autism). I also wondered whether some psychosis might be present. Although he had used marijuana problematically—possibly at the almost addiction level—it wasn't clear that his use had ever risen to the level of abuse.

Also, although his drug screening results from the last couple of months were negative for marijuana and alcohol, they were positive for amphetamine, which was expected since he was being prescribed stimulants for his ADHD. Nonetheless, the results of the drug tests couldn't tell us if he had been using his medication other than as prescribed.

And as my head was swirling with possible approaches to helping him, I was also wondering how Evan's drug use intermingled with his psychiatric status. Had marijuana and alcohol use, dating back to age fifteen, caused or contributed to his depression and anxiety? If any part of his current mix of problems was psychosis, had marijuana caused that? Or did Evan start using marijuana and alcohol in part to help calm his anxiety symptoms or as a means of self-medicating his ADHD?

Although answering these questions for any single individual can be difficult, across the population the interplay and overlap are easier to dissect, though the arrows of causation seem to go in both directions. In other words, having a mental health issue means you are more likely to develop a substance abuse problem and vice versa.

The Connections between Mental Concerns and Drug Use

Having any psychiatric diagnosis means you are more likely to have or develop a substance use disorder of some sort. According to a 2010 Substance Abuse and Mental Health Services Administration report, nearly 20 percent of adults in the United States who had any form of mental illness in the previous year also met the criteria for substance abuse or dependence during that time.[36]

Yet these figures might vastly underestimate the problem, since they describe people who have a substance use problem that rises to the level of warranting a diagnosis. They're not including the almost addicted, which means there are many more individuals with depression, anxiety, or other issues out there who are turning to illicit substances.

Again, the overlap between substance use and psychiatric illness is large. A commonly cited figure holds that among those who are seeking help for a substance use disorder, as many of 50 to 75 percent also have anxiety, depression, or some other mental health issue.[37] On the other hand, those with depression or anxiety are roughly twice as likely to have some kind of drug use disorder.[38] (As usual, one would surmise that if this figure included those who were almost addicted, the number would be greater.) In my experience working in a public general adult outpatient psychiatric clinic, I would estimate that about 70 percent of *all* my patients are misusing substances in one form or another.

The likelihood of having a coexisting substance use disorder varies from one mental health issue to another. For example, one review from 2008 found that nearly one-third of individuals with major depression also had a substance use disorder.[39] Conversely, in another large study, people with a substance use disorder were nearly five times more likely than those without a drug problem to have an affective disorder—a category that includes major depression.[40]

People with anxiety have been found to be two to four times more likely to have a substance use disorder compared to those without anxiety. And some other psychiatric problems—namely, schizophrenia, bipolar disorder, ADHD, and post-traumatic stress disorder—are related to dramatically high rates of substance use or abuse. One large study from 2006 found that 60 percent of participants with schizophrenia used drugs and 37 percent met the diagnostic criteria for a substance use disorder.[41]

Of the various psychiatric diagnoses, bipolar disorder may carry the highest risk of a substance use disorder. One 2007 study concluded that more than 40 percent of people with bipolar disorder would have a substance use disorder during their lives, and an often-cited study from 1990 put the risk of substance abuse in people with bipolar disorder at just over 60 percent.[42] Again, if these substantial figures represent people with diagnosable substance use conditions, then the actual number of individuals with bipolar disorder whose drug use falls in the gray area of almost addiction is presumably much larger.

Like these other conditions, ADHD is also associated with a significantly increased risk of illicit drug use. The correlation is quite high, and it begins in adolescence and persists into adulthood. A 2011 study that followed kids and teens for ten years into adulthood found that having a diagnosis of ADHD

Risks of Substance Use and Mental Health Issues in Military Personnel

In 2008, the US military surveyed active-duty personnel about their health and substance use, while also performing a basic screen for depression, anxiety, and PTSD. More than 28,000 service personnel responded.[43] Given the way the survey was written, it's not possible to know whether use that was problematic was in the almost range or instead qualified as abuse or dependence. We also can't tell to what extent substance use problems and mental health problems overlapped in any single individual. In general, though, co-occurring disorders were common. Here's a summary of what the study found.

Drug and Alcohol Use

- 20 percent drank more than five alcoholic drinks on the same occasion within the last thirty days.

- 12 percent used an illicit drug including prescription drug misuse within the last thirty days

- 2.3 percent used an illicit drug excluding prescription drug misuse within the last thirty days.

Mental Health Concerns

- 27 percent reported perceiving "a lot" of stress at work in the last twelve months.

- 17.6 percent reported perceiving "a lot" of stress in the family.

- 14.2 percent screened positive for anxiety and needed further evaluation.

- 21.2 percent screened positive for depression and needed further evaluation.

- 10.7 percent screened positive for PTSD and needed further evaluation.

- 4.6 percent had seriously considered suicide within the past year.

- 2.2 percent had attempted suicide within the last year.

was associated with a 47 percent higher risk of having a later substance use disorder.[44]

It's easy to speculate that a great percentage of these individuals may in fact be self-medicating their ADHD (Evan's history indicated that he may have been using his prescribed stimulant medications to get high, rather than for their intended effect). But to my knowledge, no clear data have been found to conclude this definitively. Regardless, among adolescents with ADHD, a key ingredient for developing a substance use disorder is to have a conduct disorder, which seems to play a role in the development of the drug problem.

Combat veterans, who are at risk of post-traumatic stress disorder, are another group that is very susceptible to concurrent substance use disorders and mental illness. One 2011 study found that veterans with bipolar disorder and schizophrenia were at especially high risk of also having a substance use disorder.[45]

A Closer Look at Mental Health Issues and Drug Use in Adolescents

Among teenagers and even preteens entering adolescence, the link between substance use and mental health problems—in both of the directions addressed above—might be even stronger than is the case for adults. One study, for example, found that among 359 adolescents evaluated in a psychiatric outpatient clinic, 11 percent met the criteria for a substance use disorder as identified by parental input. The researchers found that the onset of psychopathology—the mental problem—usually preceded the substance use by a year or more.[46]

A recently published European study found that 66 to 75 percent of teens with depressive symptoms used alcohol, and

19 to 29 percent used drugs (the numbers varied between boys and girls). These figures were significantly higher than for adolescents without symptoms of depression. Similarly, teens with symptoms of an eating disorder were also at significantly higher risk of using illicit drugs (22 to 32 percent of these teens did so).[47]

An older study that examined 226 adolescents who needed inpatient care for substance use disorders found that a whopping 82 percent met the criteria for at least one psychiatric diagnosis and that 74 percent met the criteria for two or more psychiatric diagnoses. Of these adolescents, 61 percent had a mood disorder, 54 percent had a conduct disorder, and 43 percent had an anxiety disorder.[48] This study and others like it suggest that the incidence of mental health disorders among adolescents who abuse substances is far higher than it is for adults. Of course, developmental factors play a role here as well, and we'll talk more about that in chapter 7.

Presuming that the ranks of the almost addicted are much larger than those who have diagnosable substance-use conditions, you can assume that the total number of adolescents who are at risk of almost addiction is substantially larger than the numbers cited in the studies mentioned here.

Adolescents who abuse drugs are usually defying and breaking more rules in order to do so than adults are. For example, adolescents are more likely than adults to lie and steal to pay for their drug use. Plus, teens often have to defy their parents' rules when using drugs, an issue not at play for most adults. Almost of necessity, then, these adolescents are greater risk-takers and are prone to more psychopathology compared with adult drug users.

Also, a thirteen-year-old child who is trying marijuana for the first time is taking far more worrisome actions than a twenty-three-year-old adult who's making an initial exploration of pot. Although using drugs at an early age does not confirm a psychiatric illness in and of itself, doing so is strongly correlated with having a diagnosable mental health disorder. Plus, many of the behaviors often associated with using drugs, such as lying and stealing, are criteria used in diagnosing conduct disorder among youths and antisocial personality disorder among adults.

The long and short of it is that numerous studies show that adolescents seeking treatment for drug use have dramatically high chances of also having a variety of mental health issues. Parents whose children have mood, behavioral, or other mental or emotional concerns would be wise to keep their antennae out for almost addiction in their kids.

So Which Condition Causes the Other?

Time and again, I've seen the coexistence of substance abuse and psychiatric illness that these researchers have observed. The presence of one condition predicts that the other will show up, too.

But does this say anything about causation (that is, if one disorder actually predisposes someone to develop the other)? The answer is likely yes, that there is some causation in both directions. As noted earlier, smoking pot even a handful of times in your life may bump up your risk of schizophrenia by 70 percent. Smoking marijuana more than fifty times may make you six times more likely to develop this life-changing disease.[49]

Conversely, having a mental health disorder can lead to

substance use as the individual attempts to self-medicate.

Nevertheless, in any particular person, it's often impossible to determine which disorder caused which. Knowing the order in which the problems became apparent can be informative, but even that is not enough to lead physicians to state with certainty that one caused the other.

In Evan's case, his ADHD diagnosis came before he ever used substances. If he had never developed ADHD, would he have still turned toward marijuana and alcohol? One has no way of knowing, of course. Also, given that both marijuana and alcohol are depressants and their use can lead to depression and anxiety, did they cause his psychiatric symptoms to arise, or would they have developed anyway, even if he'd remained completely clean through his teens and twenties?

At some point, it doesn't really matter. What is important is treating or solving the problem at hand. For someone with "only" almost addiction, this means solving the drug problem; this is important for many reasons, including the need to avoid any subsequent mental health issues that could arise from the drug use. For someone with only a mental health issue, this means relieving symptoms of that problem; again, this is necessary for many reasons besides wanting to head off possible drug use. And if someone shows up in my office with a mental health concern and almost addiction, it's vital that we find solutions to *both*.

Before leaving this discussion of "what causes what," I want to touch on a question about ADHD that may be on the minds of some readers: "Wait . . . psychiatrists and other doctors are putting kids with ADHD on stimulant drugs and apparently these drugs have enough kick that some people want to use them recreationally. Isn't it possible that the ADHD medications put kids at higher risk of developing almost addiction or other substance use problems?"

That's a valid concern, since nearly three million children and teens were being treated with medication for ADHD in 2007.[50] However, numerous studies over the years have concluded that there is "no compelling evidence that stimulant treatment of children with ADHD leads to an increased risk for substance experimentation, use, dependence, or abuse by adulthood."[51]

It's even possible that treating ADHD with medications helps protect kids from later drug use. One 2008 study followed 114 kids with ADHD for five years, until they were sixteen years old on average; 94 of them had been treated with stimulant medications. The researchers found no increased risk of substance use disorders linked to stimulant medications—and in fact, they found that kids who took these medications were 73 percent less likely to have a substance use disorder.[52] Of course, this study was looking at diagnosable disorders and not almost addiction, but it's reasonable to expect they'd go hand in hand here (the kids who took stimulant medications for their ADHD were also less likely to smoke cigarettes).

Two Problems Are Harder to Treat Than One

So it's clear that having a substance use disorder increases the chance of developing a psychiatric illness and, conversely, having a mental health disorder makes it more likely that someone will abuse a drug in some fashion, which includes becoming almost addicted. The net result is that a lot of people are dealing with both problems. And, as I've already mentioned, when both conditions are present, the prognosis for treating either successfully is poorer than if the individual had only one issue. This has been shown in study after study.

Furthermore, people with both mental health issues and substance problems face greater hardships across almost every arena of life. Poverty is more common in those with both conditions. So is homelessness. The risks of either being assaulted or assaulting someone else increase. The odds of committing suicide rise as well. The risks of accidental death or death by homicide go up. And the likelihood of engaging in high-risk behaviors in general—like having unprotected sex or otherwise taking chances with one's health—also increases, so that illness rates among them are also higher. The list goes on and on.[53]

The repercussions of combining drugs with a mood or emotional problem are massive, but I can almost hear the person with almost addiction objecting, "I don't use enough drugs to worry about being a homicide victim. That's something an addict faces. And okay, I'm a little depressed here and there, but come on. . . ."

This is a fair response, but I'd nonetheless like to point out that the combination of mental health problems and substance use that goes untreated doesn't bode well for anyone's future happiness. Combining mild depression or anxiety with almost addiction may not put you at as high of a risk for unhappiness as someone would have with a serious psychiatric condition and a heavy-duty drug problem. But if your mind, mood, or focus is already working at a somewhat limited capacity, tossing even an occasional illicit drug into the mix is going to further hamper your ability to live a content, productive life.

Looking for the Signs of Self-Medication

Why should you explore whether you're self-medicating a mental health issue with occasional drug use (or a loved one is doing so)? The answer to this question is easy: self-medicating is a bad idea because there are so many better and safer ways to treat these problems than with drugs that are potentially dangerous, usually illegal, and poorly regulated at best. (An interesting personal note: the "self-medication hypothesis"

Time to Get Professional Help?

If you experience any of the following symptoms of mental health issues, then it's probably time to get professional help:

- Persistent sadness or crying
- Anxiety beyond what is reasonable for a situation
- Excessive irritability/anger
- Difficulty paying attention or staying focused
- Apathy/not caring about things that are usually important to you
- Not being able to carry out basic functions
- Thinking about suicide or having thoughts that it'd be better not to be alive
- Psychotic symptoms, such as a feeling that you're losing touch with reality, seeing things that aren't there, or hearing voices in your head
- Feeling like you can't control your reactions to events, especially things that previously didn't bother you
- Feeling so good that you think nothing bad could ever happen to you

was first articulated several decades ago by one of my former teachers, Harvard Medical School professor Edward Khantzian.) While you're covering up mental health problems with illicit drugs, you're missing opportunities to deal with them in a more effective manner—while exposing your health and your lifestyle to all the threats that almost addiction presents. The most obvious safer alternative is to seek help from a mental health professional.

While not all legitimate psychiatric medications are uniformly safe either, this approach does ensure that a trained professional is evaluating your mental health symptoms and watching out for your safety. A professional is certainly more objective than a person who is almost addicted (or the person's friends who also use drugs) for assessing safety and risks. And following the advice of a mental health professional is surely safer than self-treating with illicit substances.

If I were in the shoes of someone who was regularly using drugs, and I was beginning to question that use, the first thing I'd do would be to give some honest thought to whether I might be self-medicating depression, anxiety, or other symptoms with my drug use. If the answer wasn't completely clear just by considering this question, I'd ask myself a few more:

• The first time I used a drug, how did it make me feel?
• Did I immediately feel as if my problems were alleviated?
• Did I feel calmer than I'd ever felt?
• Did I feel, as some drug users mention, "the way I was meant to be"?
• Have I ever been diagnosed with depression, anxiety, ADHD, PTSD, or any other mental health issue?

- Have I ever suspected that I have symptoms of any of these disorders?

- Has a close relative ever had symptoms of a mental health disorder such as depression, anxiety, ADHD, PTSD, or schizophrenia?

Answering yes to any of these questions suggests at the very least that you or the person you care about may be using drugs to self-medicate.

Another red flag is this: if you've ever taken psychiatric medications and felt better on them, but then stopped them for whatever reason (maybe you didn't like taking them or suffered from side effects) and the illicit drugs you are now using produce similar good feelings, then you might be self-medicating.

One more sign of possible self-medication is when someone craves getting high in order to relax. Although it might seem that a lot of drug use is done for the purpose of relaxing, actually only a subset of users will cite relaxation as a goal. As a result, the need for drug use to relax is a warning sign of self-medication, and it suggests the potential for greater or more problematic abuse among people with almost addiction.

At this point, I'd like to address the "but pot is natural, man" argument that I hear with some regularity. When I've encouraged people who use drugs to seek help for their mental health issues, especially when it appeared that they might be self-medicating their symptoms with drugs, more than a few marijuana fans have responded that they'd rather use a natural substance like marijuana than pollute their bodies with chemicals made by pharmaceutical companies.

Although I am critical of many practices in the pharmaceutical industry, almost without fail I'd rather see someone who has a bothersome psychiatric illness taking medications for it than not and continuing to live in pain or self-medicating. Why psychiatric drugs instead of illicit ones?

First, they are legal. The average person who's depressed or anxious isn't going to feel happier or calmer after an excursion through the legal system. Second, they are regulated and tested. Say what you will about psychiatric medications, you're going to know more about who made a medication and how it was processed than you would about a plastic bag of pot or other illicit drugs. Third, psychiatric medications are slower to kick in (with the exception of stimulant medications used for ADHD) and as such they're not as likely to cause explosions of dopamine with the resulting crash, despair, or anxiety that can follow illicit drug use.

Of course, a physician who's aware of any substance use should try to prescribe medications that don't have the potential for abuse (such as not causing euphoria), can't fetch a great price on the street, and won't lead to physical dependence.

Before leaving the topic of self-medication, I want to discuss two of the most widely used substances around the globe: caffeine and nicotine. These are legal (for adults in the case of nicotine) and are more likely to come from a reputable manufacturer than drugs bought at a party or in an alley. Still, they fall under the umbrella of substances you should carefully monitor if you have any mental health concerns.

Although caffeine can be used safely—I, for example, drink a large, strong cup of coffee daily and don't seem to have too many adverse reactions, although my family might say differently—for anyone with a tendency toward anxiety, or for anyone with ADHD who might be using it to self-medicate, caffeine should be approached with caution. My training included the dictum that caffeine is the number one cause of anxiety, period, and a classic study in 1992 illustrated the extent to which caffeine can be a significant source of anxiety for many individuals.[54]

The psychological impact of nicotine use can vary. Over the short term, its effects can be calming, but over time it seems to make depression and anxiety worse—I write *seems to* because the data are a bit conflicting on this point. Regardless, for anyone who uses tobacco and also takes psychiatric medications, tobacco may increase the speed with which certain medications are metabolized in the body, and this may necessitate taking higher doses of medication. Regular tobacco users should use caution if they find themselves suddenly deprived of tobacco, as their blood levels of the medication can then increase rapidly.

In short, it's common for people who are almost addicted to rely on their drugs—including pot, cocaine, or legal substances like cigarettes and coffee—to take the edge off their anxiety, depression, or other mental concerns. In Evan's case, I certainly wondered if his drug use provided some element of self-medication, given his strong family history of depression and anxiety, as well as the early onset of those symptoms and ADHD in his own life.

Moving from Self-Medication to Other Self-Help Steps

If you believe that you are using drugs to relieve anxiety, depression, or other mental concerns, the first thing to realize is that you can—and should—look instead to the many alternatives that are safer, more effective, and longer lasting. The goal is to take a healthy approach to eliminate or dampen your pain and suffering. This doesn't only involve making an appointment with a psychiatrist and perhaps trying psychiatric medications. Many of your options are steps that you can take on your own.

Get More Sleep

Proper sleep is essential for mental well-being. When you're tired, you're less able to maintain your focus. It's easier to feel overwhelmed and make bad decisions. And, if you have a tendency to use stimulant drugs, feeling fatigued might trigger you to look for an illicit pick-me-up. After your high and subsequent crash, you're feeling worse than when you started.

Most sleep problems can be solved by following the well-traversed rules of sleep hygiene, which include the following:

- Avoid exciting or stressful activities before bed. Save your bill paying, horror movies, and arguments with your family for a different time.

- Use your bedroom for sleeping and sex only. Don't make it the family hangout spot or the place where you work on your laptop or watch TV.

- Create a relaxing pre-bedtime routine, like taking a shower or trading backrubs with your partner. (But don't use illicit drugs or alcohol to help send you off to dreamland. They can actually interfere with quality sleep.)

- Go to bed and get up at the same time every day, weekends too.

- Avoid large meals, caffeine, and tobacco in the hours before bedtime.

- Keep your bedroom cool, dark, and quiet.

Exercise

As an avid long-distance runner and biker, I'm a huge believer in exercise for alleviating symptoms of depression and anxiety. In fact, getting regular exercise might be the single best thing someone can do for depression. Although the research is less convincing about the positive effects of exercise on anxiety, some data support it[55] and, anecdotally, I have had many patients tell me that exercise helps with their anxiety. My advice to patients is to exercise hard enough to work up a sweat for thirty minutes at a time at least five times per week.

Clean Up Your Diet

Eating properly—which means a diet rich in fresh fruits, nuts, and vegetables with minimal junk food, fast food, and other processed foods—is extremely helpful in maintaining a clear head. For example, research is now illustrating that eating a Mediterranean diet can improve symptoms of depression and anxiety. Again, this means making fruits, vegetables, nuts, whole grains, and low-fat dairy the foundation of your diet, not just the occasional healthy item you toss into your body.

Eating and exercise have been shown in animals to boost levels of dopamine in the brain. The downside of this is that eating anything—including so-called comfort food—probably boosts dopamine levels, so it's important to be careful about the kinds of food you eat.[56]

For an experiment in the other direction, Morgan Spurlock's experience can offer a useful lesson. After thirty days of eating nothing but McDonald's food in his film *Super Size Me*—and saying yes to super-sized portions whenever he was asked—he experienced sexual dysfunction and depression, in addition to a twenty-four-pound weight gain that got him lots of media attention.

Try to eat small meals and snacks often through the day, and avoid sugary foods that send your blood sugar skyrocketing and then crashing. Doing so will help keep your blood sugar on a more even keel and smooth out big dips that can leave you feeling fatigued and groggy.

Will eating a natural diet magically restore a healthy mental balance? Of course not, but it will certainly be more likely to help you than a diet heavy in junk foods.

Take Medications as Directed

In my psychiatric practice, many of my patients do not take their medications as prescribed. Antidepressants do not work effectively unless they are taken daily. Many of the antianxiety medications work terrifically, but many people will take more than prescribed in an attempt to feel *even better* and will then often run out before they are able to obtain a refill. Inevitably, when people go off these medications like this, they feel far worse than they ever did before starting the medication.

Stay Socially Active

Being in social settings keeps you connected to a web of people who might care about you, it keeps you from being alone with your thoughts so much, and it keeps your brain active with outside stimulation. Although being social may not be what you'd most like to do, when you're feeling depressed or worried, it's important to get out of your home on a regular basis.

Evan's Outcome

Since Evan began using drugs as a teenager, even his sporadic use may have increased his risk of developing a psychotic disorder, and it could have upped his chances of a mood disorder or anxiety disorder.

The disconnect he had with the rest of the world could have been psychotic, and I wondered if he had that sense of distance before he first used marijuana. If he were already vulnerable to having psychiatric illness before ever using marijuana, the pot certainly might have increased his chance of developing such a disorder. At our initial meeting, I did not see any significant signs of depression or anxiety, which might have been due to the effectiveness of the antidepressant medication he was taking (antidepressants work equally well for both depression and anxiety).

Since he was apparently clean when I met him, I encouraged him to continue steering clear of all substances of abuse. If the flatness I witnessed in him represented the early stages of schizophrenia, then staying clean was essential for minimizing the risk of whatever changes might lie ahead. In the two years he remained under my care, Evan continued to test negative for substances of abuse and remained free of any significant depression or anxiety, and he ultimately reenrolled in college.

By not living life in almost addiction and by taking his medications as prescribed, Evan would avoid the combination of two mind-altering problems that often work in tandem to destroy people's well-being. But if he ever began self-medicating his problems with marijuana, his depression, anxiety, and other mental health issues could become harder to treat.

❖

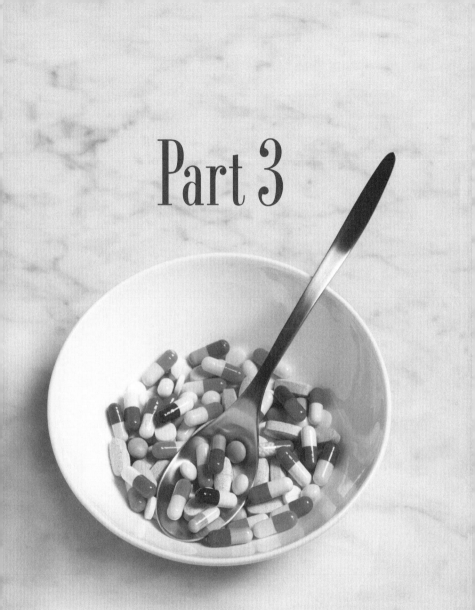

Part 3

Catching and Confronting Almost Addiction in Others

5

Recognizing an Invisible Problem

Around the world, people have gotten used to living their lives in public. Reality shows pluck people from anonymity and capture their every move with dozens of cameras. Facebook, Twitter, and other social-networking sites allow you to upload photos and share any thought that pops into your head with hundreds or thousands of friends and acquaintances.

Just a few years ago, personal and private moments might be embarrassing or even ruin one's reputation if they were revealed publicly. Nowadays, you might upload this same information or related pictures yourself and invite strangers to comment on them.

Even if you don't want people in your business, strangers can easily find your address and look at a street-side view of your home, then look up its value online. People can read about you in newspaper archives that stay online indefinitely.

Yes, it's hard to keep an important secret these days. Yet when it comes to drug use, people with almost addiction can do this very well—if they see a reason to. In some cases, almost addicted individuals are unaware that their substance use is causing any problems and so they make no effort to cover up or conceal their use. It can remain an "open" secret that their peers may see but not find unusual enough to discuss.

Those who do sense that something might be wrong with their substance use—if only because the drug is illegal—might take great pains to conceal the extent of their use. If they don't appear intoxicated around other people, and if they're not addicted and therefore don't show any physical signs of withdrawal, then without other information or reason for concern other people may not easily detect that they are almost addicted. With just a bit of effort, they can fly under their families' radar. They can conceal the signs of their drug use from even their doctors.

That's why both types of almost addicted individuals—those who don't see a problem with their drug use and those who hide it—may not raise the red flags that can lead people around them to try to help.

For my patient Gianni, drug use added to his problems for years, even though plenty of people in his life could have alerted him to his almost addiction, from his family to his health care providers.

Gianni's Story

Gianni first came to our clinic when he was twenty years old and a part-time student at a local junior college. He had just been hospitalized for overwhelming panic and depression that had driven him to the point of wanting to kill himself. Before his hospitalization, he was holed up in his bedroom, contemplating why he ought to just "get it over with," when the thought of calling 911 occurred to him.

The police arrived, and after talking with Gianni, they placed him in the backseat of a cruiser and drove him to the psychiatric emergency room for an evaluation. He stayed in the inpatient psychiatric unit for five days, where he was prescribed a daily antidepressant for his depression and anxiety and given a tranquilizer, as needed.

I met Gianni soon after he was discharged. He no longer wanted to kill himself, saying that he realized he needed to stay alive for his newborn son. But he still felt terrible, with overwhelming anxiety and depression. He had several big stressors in his life. He'd been out of work for six months, had no money, and was living with his parents. His relationship with the mother of his son was on-again, off-again, and his emotions were constantly up and down as a result. Still, his biggest concern was that the boy might not actually be his biological son.

Against this backdrop of stressors, Gianni told me that he felt severe anxiety anytime he was around others and was "paranoid" that they were looking at him and negatively judging him. He said that he often had trouble breathing, sweated constantly, and usually felt on the verge of a full-blown panic attack.

As a child, he'd been diagnosed with attention deficit disorder, which went untreated. He eventually quit school in the eleventh grade because of his inability to concentrate on his schoolwork, combined with his social phobia. He did eventually complete a GED and had recently enrolled in college. Starting at age fifteen, he had occasionally seen psychiatrists, who prescribed a number of medications for his depression and anxiety. He'd also been in therapy off and on over the years.

His parents often engaged in loud shouting matches. His father would beat Gianni and his siblings regularly after he'd been drinking, sometimes for no apparent reason. Not surprisingly, all of the kids had problems with anxiety, and several were addicted to marijuana. Gianni said that as his mother got older, she eventually sought treatment for anxiety, as had her own mother.

He had smoked marijuana sporadically since age fifteen. He considered his current marijuana use "low." Although he would smoke anywhere from once a month to once a week, he hadn't smoked in several months. At sixteen, he tried cocaine for the first time and said he had used it a total of ten times when I met with him. He said he'd abused Percocet for a few weeks after having an emergency appendectomy when he was eighteen, but stopped when his supply ran out. He also tried Ecstasy a handful of times over the course of a couple of months when he was nineteen. He liked the way it made him feel, but he had a terrible crash when he was coming off it.

When I met Gianni, he was on probation. He had been arrested twice, once for trespassing and another time for assault and battery. He offered a lengthy explanation about why both of these charges were unjust. Gianni never thought that his substance use had caused any trouble in his life, with the exception of the way he felt while coming off Ecstasy.

He didn't see a link between the drugs and his hospitalization, his arrests, his rocky relationship with his girlfriend, or his depression and anxiety. His family had never confronted him about his drug use. His doctors had never dug into the role that drugs could be playing in his mental and emotional health problems either.

But as I got to know him, I suspected that his drug use could certainly be a factor in all of these problems.

Why Drugs May Not Seem Like a Problem to the Almost Addicted

When people have done well socially and financially, it's easy to see why they might not consider their drug use to be problematic. After all, if you are getting promotions at work and your friends and colleagues regularly praise you, how on earth could a little cocaine or marijuana a few times a week pose a problem?

It can be much harder to recognize almost addicted behavior in individuals who are successful. After all, the old adage says "You can't argue with success," and to a large extent this is true. Most people don't have the audacity to tell a self-made millionaire or a high-flying attorney that he might have a problem that is keeping him from reaching his full potential. In addition to having social or financial success, these individuals are often more intelligent than average. And smarter people often have to fall further before a problem becomes apparent to others or they reach out for help.

One British study found that when physicians had drug dependency—which is a problem that goes well beyond almost addiction—problematic drug use had occurred for about six and a half years on average before the physician sought help for the problem.[57] The reason for this may be that if someone is fairly skilled and adept at navigating the world (and making the world conform to her own wishes), she is going to be able to conceal a problem longer. Similarly, I've noticed that when senior professionals and executives, who often have spectacularly high IQs, begin to show signs of dementia, they often have to sink well below their prior level of functioning before the problem becomes apparent to others.

In some cases, the people surrounding a successful individual might be able to pick up on a problem like almost addiction. On the other hand, the individual may be able to conceal the sometimes subtle effects of the almost addiction on his mood, focus, schedule, and bank account.

In other settings, a person who has struggled with any number of obstacles and missed opportunities in his childhood and present life, as Gianni had, may find it easy to blame any of these factors for his failures and unreached goals, rather than his occasional drug use. And so may the people around him. After all, when someone has abusive parents, lack of education, nightmares of childhood traumas, no job, and a disintegrating relationship, some drug use may not seem like a leading source of hindrance.

Many other elements in a person's life could also make almost addiction seem like a relatively minor or nonexistent concern.

First, drug use that pushes the boundaries of acceptability can seem normal if many people around the individual also use drugs. Along these lines, I have heard many, many teenagers and young adults—and more than a few middle-aged adults—tell me that every person they know uses drugs. In any given social group, if every single person is using a drug, how can doing so be considered either abnormal or problematic, especially if some of these same individuals are deeply respected and admired by the group? If you grew up in England, driving on the left side of the road seems perfectly normal because that's all you've ever known.

Almost addiction can also be overlooked if just a few people in one's surroundings make drug use seem cool and part of an enviable lifestyle. If the people around you who have great looks, wear hip clothing, and date beautiful people keep their position in society even though they snort a little coke during the week, couldn't that serve as an endorsement for drug use?

I knew someone just like this when I was in college. He was smart, handsome, a little exotic in appearance, and unafraid to ingest any drug that came his way. Although he didn't use drugs daily or even every week, everyone knew that he was game for anything. He was brilliant and always excelled academically, and no one would have suggested that he had a problem with drugs. Nevertheless, he later progressed to a substance abuse problem that led him to start attending AA meetings.

Yet another reason why some people with almost addiction are overlooked is because they are never looked over at all; that is, some are loners who keep to themselves. If you rarely venture outside of your home or open your life up to other people, you're going to have fewer chances to learn from others, or to reveal to others, that your drug use is a problem.

Finally, when it comes to looking in a mirror and seeing yourself clearly and without blinders (which is the kind of observation necessary to fully recognize that you have a problem), humans have remarkably cloudy vision. Research has repeatedly shown that when considering matters close to home, people are simply not able to behave rationally and without bias.

So if you're frustrated that a friend or loved one isn't seeing her own almost addiction, one or more of these explanations may be the reason.

Factors That Can Make Almost Addiction Invisible to the User

- **Success.** If you're one of society's "winners" based on your accomplishments, career, luck, or smarts, it may be hard for others to attribute a quality not associated with winning to you (for example, drug use).

- **Coolness.** One element of appearing "cool" can be a willingness to take risks. Drug use is one type of risk-taking behavior. And when people perceive you as a cool or hip person they want to be like, they probably aren't going to point out a shortcoming they perceive, such as drug use.

- **Reclusiveness.** If you don't give people any insight into your personal choices, they're not going to have a chance to observe issues that could be causing you problems.

- **High intelligence.** If you're a smart person, you're likely better at concealing your drug use. Not only may you be more discreet about your use and clever about coming up with alibis and cover stories, your smarts may come with the success that can discourage others from confronting you.

- **Surroundings.** If most of your friends and family use drugs—especially if they use them heavily—it's less likely that the people who know you best would suggest that you have a problem with drugs. In addition, the situation will make it easy for you to say, "I don't have a drug problem compared to my friend Eddie, or my friend Cindy, or my aunt Linda."

Why Family Members and Friends Might Miss an Almost Addiction

There are many reasons why other people who ostensibly know those with an almost addiction best—their family—can also miss a problem.

The first and perhaps easiest explanation is that any complications from the drug use have not presented themselves to the family members. In other words, none of them has witnessed it directly. I have certainly seen my share of people who are almost addicted whose use triggered no outward warning signs. I have even seen a number of people whose drug consumption was so secretive and well concealed that short of a urine test or direct observation, parents and spouses would have virtually no reason to suspect drug use.

It's not surprising that people who are almost addicted can carry on their drug use below the awareness of their families, since people with true addictions can as well. I think back to my work with Chrissie, who had a true opiate addiction and used a dosage of OxyContin large enough to kill an entire family. Her habit was so all-consuming that when the police finally caught her after a year and a half of use, they assumed she had to be dealing drugs because otherwise she'd have been dead. But until she was caught, nobody around her—including her husband and numerous co-workers—had any suspicions whatsoever. If she could get away with hiding this elephant of a drug habit, people who are almost addicted can find their less frequent drug use quite easy to conceal.

But let's suppose that the drug use should be visible to anyone who was nearby. Even when that's the case, it's still remarkably easy for loved ones to convince themselves that no problem exists. Such denial is a basic human impulse, especially when it comes to people you care about deeply. It is all too easy to will oneself into ignorance about possible drug use, since people generally want to see their loved ones in a favorable light and may minimize or be blind to problems that are right in front of their eyes. (I have told people many times that if my mother saw me shoot someone at point-blank range without provocation, it would take only a few minutes for her to convince herself that I didn't pull the trigger or, at worst, it was purely in self-defense.)

This is the way people's minds work. They rally around those they love. They are not rational about some things even when they try to be, especially when love or other emotional hot-button matters are at stake. How could they see a problem in close family members when they are naturally predisposed toward seeing their good qualities?

So if you feel bad because you've suspected that a loved one is dealing with almost addiction but you kept your concerns to yourself, or because you now realize that you've been missing obvious signs of a problem, it's perfectly understandable.

Conversely, if you are the one who is almost addicted and your family hasn't questioned you or confronted you about it (yet), don't assume that they're quietly approving your choices. Any number of other reasons could explain their silence.

Beyond simply missing an almost addiction, family members can also aid and abet almost addiction in various ways. A common way that families respond to any form of drug use, from occasional marijuana smoking to a full-blown heroin addiction, is to remain silent. Unlike the person who is in denial, family members who keep silent might see the problem

—perhaps even being painfully aware of it—but simply choose to say nothing.

Maybe they are afraid of the conflict that might ensue if they were to bring up the obvious. Perhaps they don't want to get their loved one into trouble, and they feel like they are making the situation better with their silence. Maybe they don't know the right way to bring up the issue. Maybe they're afraid the almost addicted relative will point out their own shortcomings or accuse them of bad parenting and causing the drug use in the first place.

Family members can help facilitate and prolong an almost addiction. They can provide money and other material support to help the drug use continue. Some actually hand out money as the individual is heading out the door to buy drugs. But the funding may not be so obvious. If someone who is spending his cash on drugs is constantly short when it comes to rent or groceries, then paying for his rent or food is almost like directly paying for the drugs. That's because when someone else is taking care of these needs, the almost addicted individual is shielded from the consequences of spending money on drugs instead of essentials.

Because substance use runs in families and is mirrored within families, other drug users in the family can inspire the almost addicted person to keep going. Past or present drug use within the group creates a tone and a culture in which drug use is acceptable or even expected, which can make a family member feel that it's easier and more normal to use drugs, too. This is yet another reason why spouses or families may be hesitant to confront someone who is almost addicted: they don't want to hear about their own past or present drug or alcohol use.

Factors That Can Make Almost Addiction Invisible to Families

- **Help with money.** Paying the almost addicted person's bills is a common way that families unwittingly support a loved one's drug use. If the individual has a place to live, a car, and a regular schedule that this financial assistance allows, others may be less likely to suspect a drug problem. If a loved one repeatedly loses jobs or is constantly in need of money, you should consider drug use as a possible reason. If an individual is known to be using drugs, then families can help address the problem by withholding money rather than handing it over.

- **Denial.** Denial is a basic human impulse, especially when it comes to a loved one. It is all too easy to will oneself into ignorance about possible drug use, especially when you are talking about almost addiction, when the hints can be subtle.

- **Silence.** This is a closely related cousin of denial. Unlike the person who is in denial, the loved one who keeps silent might see the problem—perhaps even be profoundly aware of the problem—but simply chooses to not speak. Often family members don't speak up because they think that not causing trouble for a family member is the best course of action. Almost always, this course actually worsens problems related to the almost addiction.

- **Other drug use in the family.** If other people in the family use drugs, it is much more likely that any particular member of that family will also be using. When drugs are more common, family members may not realize that drug use is unhealthy and illegal, or they may feel like hypocrites if they speak up.

Why Health Professionals Might Miss an Almost Addiction

Watch a season of the TV show *House*—or episodes of medical shows featuring real-life physicians—and you might think that doctors can catch any medical problem, no matter how mysterious or obscure.

However, Gianni had ventured into the health care system many times before he met me. He had talked to all sorts of gatekeepers at hospitals and other health facilities, including nurses, doctors, and mental health professionals. But I don't know that any of them expressed much concern for his drug use.

Doctors and other medical professionals overlook almost addiction all the time. They might miss or even ignore the problem for many reasons. For example, they may feel that their patients won't follow any recommendations they'd make about their drug use anyway. Or they may not have the expertise to detect a subtle drug problem or counsel patients about it effectively.

But of all the reasons why a primary care provider might fail to recognize or acknowledge someone who is almost addicted —much less ask screening questions about substance use—a common one is that health care professionals perpetually feel like they do not have enough time to do so. If they do uncover a drug problem, many may not know what to do about it (while worrying that trying to find a solution will eat up a big chunk of their day).[58] Most primary care clinicians around the world feel squeezed by time pressure and productivity requirements, so doing any investigation or counseling outside of their basic routine with a patient can become overwhelming.

One survey of 1,082 general internists, family physicians, obstetricians and gynecologists, and psychiatrists assessed their practices regarding illicit drug use and found that roughly one-third of respondents did not regularly ask new patients about drug use. Among those who did diagnose substance abuse, 55 percent reported that they routinely offered a referral for treatment and 15 percent reported that they did not take action.[59]

This frequent lack of drug screening isn't all that surprising. Research found that if primary care physicians completed all of the recommended preventive services and screens on each of their patients, a doctor with typical patients would have to spend more than seven hours of every working day just completing these duties. That leaves no time for dealing with a patient's illness, no time for talking about feeling sad because of a recent breakup, and certainly no time to inquire about the nuances of substance use in someone who is not obviously addicted or heavily abusing drugs.[60]

If physicians do have time to dig into a patient's substance use and their effort turns up information that actually requires counseling and action of some sort, doctors will need to spend even more time intervening or referring the patient for treatment elsewhere. Another reason many clinicians don't broach this topic with their patients is that they don't believe materials are available to help the patient address the problem.[61]

Similarly, some clinicians don't dig too deeply into drug use because they believe, wrongly, that there is no hope for patients who are misusing substances, because they are unwilling to change. On that note, my feeling is that asthma, diabetes, and heart disease can appear equally difficult to treat, and yet only a completely incompetent primary care physician would shy away from doing everything possible for such patients. Why should problematic drug use be any different?

Another factor some physicians cite, when asked why they don't do more for their patients who misuse drugs, is that they don't get reimbursed adequately for doing so. Although this fact might seem crass to some readers, these doctors do have a point. Physicians often have a business to keep going, and most are overworked. During an action-packed day, they essentially have to pick and choose where they should focus their attention. If one visit pays $100 and another pays little but costs precious time, which way is the physician likely to go?

But beneath these possible reasons for overlooking almost addiction, I'd surmise that a deeper psychological issue might be at play. Health care professionals may see their patients who are well-spoken, successful professionals as peers—even if they are almost addicted. When this happens, the clarity that health care professionals might otherwise have can be obscured. They might, therefore, subconsciously avoid thinking about problematic behavior in someone whom they view, in part, like themselves.

When doctors fail to catch a case of almost addiction, it presents a missed opportunity for the patient to obtain help for a serious problem. Patients may conclude, "If the doctor doesn't see this as a problem, why should I?"

A term known as *medicalization* has come to define many people's everyday lives in countries around the world. Medicalization occurs when a concern or symptom that used to be regarded as a common element of human existence becomes seen instead as a medical problem that a doctor needs to treat.

These include a long list of issues including menopause, hair loss, premenstrual syndrome (PMS), and erectile dysfunction. Medicalized problems aren't necessarily a sign that society has become too sensitive to finding disease wherever it turns. Some of these issues do deserve medical attention and treatment, such as alcoholism and addiction, which are now recognized as a disease rather than viewed as a personal weakness, as in the past.

But in a time when health care providers have become the authority for handling many personal and social problems, any issue they overlook can seem trivial by default. After all, patients take their moles, lumps, and coughs to the doctor every day to see if the symptom is a cause for action. And if the doctor doesn't think it's a problem, you may be able to easily push it out of your mind. The same goes with almost addiction.

Conversely, if a society doesn't consider almost addiction to be a medical problem that requires treating, an overworked and understaffed health care field may not feel the need to make an issue of it, either.

So if your loved one uses the gambit that "Hey, my doctor never asked me whether I'm using drugs," or "I told my doctor I smoke pot on occasion and she didn't make a big deal about it," that's no reason to drop your own interest in the matter.

Having said all this, people who are almost addicted should expect their doctor to take almost addiction seriously if they go to the doctor seeking help for the problem. We'll talk about how people who are almost addicted can get help from doctors and mental health providers in chapter 9.

Making an Unseen Problem Visible

For people who have been keeping an almost addiction either expertly camouflaged or openly practiced yet unacknowledged, the following steps can help put the issue on the table so you

**Factors That Can Make Almost Addiction
Invisible to Health Care Providers**

- **Lack of time.** Doctors pick their battles every day. If their schedule is filled with urgent matters like chest pain, out-of-control diabetes, or suicidal thoughts, a subtle problem like almost addiction in an otherwise healthy patient is not likely to attract attention.

- **Lack of training.** Many doctors simply may not know what to do about drug use that hasn't reached the addiction stage.

- **Lack of optimism.** Some doctors may think that the patient is going to be unwilling to change, so it's not worth putting a lot of effort into counseling.

- **No reimbursement.** While the public may like to think that health care providers work purely for benevolent reasons, financial pressure may affect their decisions in many cases. If they're not going to be adequately paid for doing a job—like sniffing out and treating almost addiction—they may not make this task a priority.

can begin to discuss it and resolve it. Although I'll delve more deeply into ways to handle almost addiction with a loved one in the next chapter, the recommendations that follow are a good place to start.

Open a Dialogue with Your Loved One

If you're reading this book on behalf of someone else, find a good time to raise the topic of almost addiction. Tell your loved one you're concerned that she may be using drugs and suffering negative consequences as a result. Explain what you've learned from the book so far: that people from all walks of life can become almost addicted and that drug use can cause life-altering problems even for people who are steadily employed and are meeting all of their family and other obligations.

Inform this person that even if she denies the problem, you're going to remain concerned as long as you feel like she is indeed almost addicted. The problem is not going to become invisible to you as long as she continues to use drugs.

Discuss Other Drug Use in Your Family

If other people in your family are using drugs or have done so in the past, now is a good time to discuss that, too. It will help put your loved one's use into context. A frank discussion about this wider pattern may help shed more light on why your loved one has become almost addicted. This better understanding of your family's relationship to substances may help lead to solutions as well.

Bring in a Doctor's Help

Urge your loved one to make an appointment to discuss the drug use with a doctor or mental health provider. Physicians are accustomed to hearing stories of people's questionable behaviors and decisions, and the doctor has almost certainly talked to patients about poorer or more unusual decisions than this possible almost addiction.

Although many primary care doctors may not go out of their way to uncover their patients' drug use, it's a different matter when a patient makes an appointment specifically to discuss it. In these cases, a good doctor will sit up, take an interest in the problem, and offer some kind of intervention to help solve it. Doctors are accustomed to helping people find the motivation to change all kinds of health-affecting behaviors, including smoking and drinking. If stress or depression may be playing a role in the drug use, the doctor can likely prescribe a legitimate medication that can address these factors or at the very least can refer the individual to a mental health professional.

If your loved one can't launch this conversation with a health professional, urge him to bring along a confidant who can do so (perhaps you!). A patient I've been seeing for fifteen years recently informed me that he has been abusing the stimulant medication that I prescribed him. He couldn't quite tell me himself (I suspect because he likes me, respects me, and feels bad for having duped me) that he was abusing these medications, but he could allow his wife to do so. It can be quite difficult to openly and honestly assess one's own drug use and set a path for change. A good doctor won't judge your loved one for having a drug problem or make her feel guilty or ashamed.

Gianni's Outcome

Like many people who are almost addicted, Gianni initially did not have any concerns about his drug use. In our very first meeting, I planted the seed of an idea that even his sporadic drug use might be making his psychological symptoms worse. Since he constantly talked about how much he wanted a job in order to make money and feel good about himself as a man, I emphasized the financial cost of using drugs, since drug use is usually not an inexpensive endeavor.

Earning decent money would allow him to move out of his parents' home and be a good father to his son as well as a positive role model for him, he said. Knowing that Gianni desired these things allowed me to use a motivational interviewing approach to point out the space between his drug use and his desires to be a responsible man, a good father, and a valuable employee.

I also pointed out the concern that his illegal drug use could get him arrested and put him significantly further away from meeting all of his goals.

Gianni was smart and keenly observant of others. Because of this, he knew that using drugs was an impediment to reaching his goals—which included completing junior college and obtaining steady work—and we discussed this discrepancy. But even for users who are not addicted, drugs tug strongly, and stopping them is difficult. Gianni's difficulty in stopping was rooted in part among the friends he kept, most of whom used drugs regularly and none of whom saw any problem with it. Most of them, Gianni knew, were headed nowhere in life, and he wanted to be different.

After we had worked together several years, Gianni had mostly moved on from his old friends—a common necessity for someone whose social group uses drugs—and he had almost entirely stopped using illicit drugs. He also completed his associate degree in computer science. Despite several initial disappointments in landing regular employment, he eventually got an unpaid internship at a university helping with Internet security. He felt quite lucky to have the job and knew that the university might drug test him at any time. Voilá, he entirely ceased all drug use.

When the internship ended, the university kept him on in a paid position, with solid wages and benefits. Gianni is now spending plenty of time with his son, and he's saved enough money to rent his own apartment. Although there are still numerous stresses in his life, he feels and looks better than he has in the previous five years.

His life is finally falling into place, and his newfound success is due in part to conquering his almost addiction.

■ ◆ ■

| 6 |

Confronting and Solving
a Loved One's Almost Addiction

Only rarely will the person with almost addiction confess to using drugs. Usually, the individual simply denies any drug use. This denial can come in the form of a blasé brush-off or an explosive rant.

Trying to reconcile these denials with the evidence of almost addiction that you've seen can leave you confused. Your world can be turned topsy-turvy when you aren't sure what you're seeing. The almost addicted person can say he's not using, when you've noted on multiple occasions that he's either used drugs or has shown clear signs of drug use. People who are almost addicted may go to great lengths to convince you that you can't believe what you see. As a result, being around someone who is almost addicted can be incredibly hard.

I've seen the faces of family members who were confused, dazed, and angry about a loved one's drug use, and I've dealt with their question: What's a family member to do? Even though a loved one's almost addiction can make your reality hard to understand, you can take steps to cut through someone else's denial and get help both for yourself and for this person.

David's Story

David was himself a psychiatrist who was referred to me from a rehab facility where he'd spent the previous two weeks. He landed there because of a Vicodin habit, which he'd developed over a two-year period.

Although he started off almost addicted, he had progressed to daily, heavy drug use. For the last year before entering treatment, David had been writing prescriptions for himself in his cousin's name. His ruse came to an abrupt halt on one of his daily stops to the many pharmacies he visited to fill yet another Vicodin prescription.

On that particular day, the pharmacist asked David to wait a moment while he filled the prescription. Instead of filling it, the pharmacist called the police. Within a few hours, David had surrendered his license to prescribe medications, stopped practicing medicine, and instead of going to jail went directly into a detox facility for a week followed by a two-week stay in rehab.

Just how did David end up here?

David had thought about becoming a doctor for most of his childhood. He attended an excellent college, but lacked focus while he was there, partly because he'd fallen for a woman who would break his heart several times over a six-year period. In order to stay near her, he took a job after graduation landscaping for a local company. After a year of working on lawns, he became disillusioned with both his relationship and his job. His dream of becoming a doctor was reignited and he signed up at a local college for the several premed courses he lacked, excelled in them, and applied for medical school.

During the year after college, David started using cocaine on occasion. Although the times he'd drunk alcohol or smoked marijuana left him unmoved, cocaine was a completely different story. He didn't do coke often, but every time he used it he felt euphoric. The drug lifted him out of his misery and made him forget the toil of his daily work and the sadness that permeated his relationship.

During medical school, David almost entirely stopped using cocaine. He finally let go of his troubled relationship and in the midst of his third-year rotations, met a nurse, Joanna, whom he eventually married during his first year of residency. He chose psychiatry because he liked spending time with patients and hearing their stories. During his last year of residency, David and Joanna had a baby girl. His wife promptly quit her job to stay home with their daughter. David's parents and one of his siblings lived in the same town, and the extended family would get together frequently.

After the residency, David was hired at a local clinic that demanded its psychiatrists see a high volume of patients. This expectation meant he had only minimal interaction with patients, something he came to increasingly resent the longer he was there. As his new work became more and more routine, David and Joanna grew apart. With Joanna no longer working in medicine, they found that they had less in common.

As he later told the story, here he was a married father with a new career and new house . . . in other words, everything he had ever wanted. There was just one problem—he was bored. His wife no longer excited him and his work had become rote and dull.

It was against this setting that David had a minor collision while driving home from work. His knee was badly bruised and swelled rapidly. EMTs on the scene took him to a nearby emergency room for evaluation. X-rays showed that he had not fractured any bones. Without even asking for medication for the pain, David was discharged from the emergency room with a prescription for sixty tablets of Vicodin, an opiate painkiller.

Prior to taking these Vicodin tablets, David had never taken opiates. He said with the very first tablet he took, his pain diminished and he felt a good, warm sensation inside.

Although he initially used them exclusively for pain, because of how good they made him feel, he began to take them at other times. At first, his Vicodin use settled in to about once every week or two. He only used these tablets after work when nobody was around, and he said they helped him unwind and feel relaxed and good. After about six months, his use increased to one or two tablets per week. But just a short time later, he was taking Vicodin daily. He said it helped him forget about the boredom in his marriage and the hopeless feeling he had about his job.

After about three months, his supply of Vicodin was running out and the thought of not having it around made him nervous. He told his primary care doctor that he was having some residual knee pain and obtained a prescription for another thirty pills. Unlike his first prescription, he ran through this one quickly.

During his first several months of Vicodin use, I would consider David to be almost addicted. He hadn't gotten into any kind of trouble because of the drug, hadn't broken any laws to obtain it, and was acting responsibly in every facet of his life—except that he was now using the Vicodin for purposes other than it was intended.

After his second prescription ran out, and after his primary care doctor refused to give him a refill, David first planned to simply stop using the Vicodin, but that proved much more difficult both mentally and physically than he'd expected. That's when he stole his cousin's driver's license, wrote his first illicit prescription for ninety tablets of Vicodin in his cousin's name, paid cash, and in short order descended from almost addiction into full-blown addiction.

But David's story prompts this question: Could his family have noticed his problems and stepped in earlier? After all, his parents lived in the area and his wife had been a medical professional. What signs might they have overlooked?

In this chapter, I'll discuss how to recognize and cope with almost addiction among loved ones in general. Then, in the next chapter, I'll talk about special issues involved in almost addiction at both ends of the age spectrum: adolescents and young adults, and seniors.

Seeing the Signs of Almost Addiction in a Loved One

Many warning signs can tip off a family member that a loved one might be misusing drugs. Many of these are nonspecific, which is to say they don't mean that someone is definitely using drugs. They could instead be signs that other issues are going on or that the person is just having a bad day.

So if a loved one shows a single clue of those listed below, or even several of them, don't automatically assume that drugs are the culprit. Nonetheless, if you have a suspicion that someone might be using drugs, these are the hints that you should look for to assess and possibly confirm your hunch.

Here are some of the physical warning signs of drug abuse:

- **Deterioration in appearance.** This can include poor grooming or worsening personal hygiene. These signs may be less obvious in a person with almost addiction compared with someone in full-blown addiction, but you may still be able to note that something feels slightly off with the person's appearance from time to time.

- **Visible weight changes or significant changes in appetite or eating.** Some drugs may cause the person to want to eat more than usual, with marijuana being well known for this effect. Other drugs, such as heroin and other opiates, can cause a drop in appetite and weight.

- **Excessive fatigue.** When someone who is almost addicted is under the influence of a sedating or relaxing medication, she may appear sleepy. Conversely, if someone is using stimulating substances—like cocaine or amphetamines—he may seem notably fatigued when he isn't directly under the influence of the drug.

- **Sleeping much more or much less.** When people are "crashing" after being high on a stimulant, they can often sleep for extended periods of time. If you notice changes in sleeping habits, drugs could be playing a role.

- **Slurred speech.** Occasionally people slur their speech

when they are tired, but this can indicate drug use. (Of course, some people slur their speech naturally; when this occurs with people who already have a drug history, it can set off a lot of false alarms, as happened with one of my clients.)

• **Falling.** Everyone is entitled to a stumble now and then without any warning bells going off, but don't rule out drug use if falling is anything other than exceedingly rare in a young or middle-age adult.

• **Eye changes.** The use of certain drugs can cause people's pupils to change size dramatically. Cocaine or amphetamines, for example, will cause pupils to dilate and open widely, whereas opiates will cause pupils to become very small and be "pinned," as in pinpoints. Given that David was using opiates, if his family had been vigilant, they might have noticed that his pupils were frequently constricted.

• **Needle marks, bruises, or bandages.** Unless someone has a very good reason for needle marks on the inner arms (and the fairly short list of good reasons includes giving blood or getting injections of legitimate medication), your suspicion of drug use should increase dramatically if you notice these marks. Also, long sleeves on a hot day may indicate that the person is concealing needle marks.

There are also a number of behavioral changes that can indicate drug use. Like the physical signs noted above, these can serve as nonspecific warning signs.

- **Deterioration in quality of performance at work or in school.** I have seen many, many instances of people having a drop in grades exactly when they begin using marijuana or some other drug. Almost addiction can trigger this change. Yet, more often than not, when I've pointed out the correlation between drug use and the drop in performance, patients swore that the two were unrelated. However, this sign doesn't always arise. Unlike many who abuse drugs, David had not been visibly less productive at work—when the police quizzed David's workmates after he was busted, not one person in his workplace noticed any deterioration in the quality of his work, even though for the last year of his drug use he was high all day long.

- **Repeated absences from important activities.** For people who function at a high performance level at work and need to show up on time to maintain their success, this sign can be especially dramatic and important. As his drug use escalated, David had to remove himself more and more from family functions both to obtain his drug and also to use it. This is a visible sign that, in retrospect, his wife and other family members may have noticed.

- **Continual seeking of special accommodations.** If someone repeatedly asks for special treatment in some form or other, such as extra time to get here or there, it might be in order to cover up for drug use.

- **Repeated trouble getting along with others.** This occurs in part because people tend to make bad decisions while high. While under the influence, they may act selfishly and without consideration for others, which often creates conflict. It's also common for anger and the potential for violence to increase when someone begins using drugs. This can be the result of being intoxicated on stimulating drugs or being more irritable and angry when other more sedating drugs leave the system.

• **Need for more money than before.** Drugs are often expensive. Also, people who are almost addicted can make bad decisions about work that lead to job loss, thereby creating a cash-flow crisis. Furthermore, while under the influence, people may make foolish purchases that are beyond their means. For all of these reasons, money often becomes scarce when people are using, and they often resort to borrowing or stealing to get it. For example, even though he made a good living, David was running through money at a phenomenal rate since he was paying cash to fill the Vicodin prescriptions. Someone with less income might run into a financial bind even during an almost addiction.

• **Secrecy about one's whereabouts.** Given that David and his wife were somewhat disconnected from one another prior to his drug use, it was easy for him to engage in secretive behaviors. If you have a close relationship with someone who is almost addicted, the time she spends chasing down drugs (or getting high or coming down from the drug) may easily raise your concern.

• **Change in friends.** Many people use drugs with—and get them from—a certain set of friends and acquaintances. So if your loved one has a sudden shift in whom he spends time with, drugs could certainly be the explanation.

Finally, there are also a number of psychological signs that can point to possible drug use. These include the following:

- **Changes of personality.** When individuals use drugs, even occasionally, they often have a major change in personality. Many times I've sat across from parents of

---

Is My Loved One Almost Addicted?

The following material is adapted from Al-Anon, the group that helps family members sort through the issues that come with having a family member who abuses a substance.[62] The purpose of the quiz is to assess whether you are affected by the drug use (not just alcoholism) of someone in your family, a close friend, or a romantic partner.

- Do you worry about how much someone uses drugs?
- Do you have money problems because of someone else's drug use?
- Do you tell lies to cover up for someone else's drug use?
- Do you feel that if the drug user cared about you, he or she would stop using drugs to please you?
- Do you blame the user's behavior on his or her companions?
- Are plans frequently canceled or meals delayed because of the person who is using drugs?
- Do you make threats, such as "If you don't stop using, I'll leave you"?
- Are you afraid to upset this person for fear it will set off an episode of drug use?
- Have you been hurt or embarrassed by the user's behavior?

drug users who say something to the effect of "I don't recognize my child anymore."

- **Constant sadness or tearfulness.** Of course, these symptoms could indicate depression, but they might also be signs of drug use or abuse. As noted earlier in the

- Are holidays and gatherings spoiled because of drug use?
- Have you considered calling the police for help because you're physically afraid?
- Do you search for hidden drugs?
- Do you ever ride in a car with a driver who has been using drugs?
- Have you refused social invitations out of fear or anxiety?
- Do you feel like a failure because you can't control the drug use?
- Do you think that if this person stopped using drugs, your other problems would be solved?
- Do you ever threaten to hurt yourself to scare the drug user?
- Do you feel angry, confused, or depressed most of the time?
- Do you feel that no one understands your problems?

Answering yes to any of these questions means that you might have an almost addicted person in your life. Taking to heart the recommendations you've just read could help you cope with a difficult circumstance, while helping ensure that your loved one gets help before an almost addiction triggers a life-changing problem—or turns into a flat-out addiction.

book, some people may turn to drugs as a way to treat underlying depression, so drugs and depression aren't mutually exclusive. Expressions of hopelessness or worthlessness might also be depression talking, but they could also grow out of drug use.

- **Constant anxiety, mood swings, or irritability.** As with the symptoms above, these could indicate emotional or mood problems, but they might also be fallout from drug use. Or they could point to both issues. In all likelihood, David was showing mood swings during his almost addicted phase. Had his family been alert to these symptoms, they might have intervened early and prevented his eventual tailspin into full-blown addiction, with all of its costs.

- **Unprovoked anger or hostility.** This is a remarkably common aspect of drug use.

- **Lack of motivation.** Drug use can sap people's motivation in general. Marijuana in particular can make getting motivated very, very difficult. Someone who operates at a high intellectual level might show a noticeable falloff even if they're using drugs only occasionally.

- **Isolation.** Often when individuals begin using drugs, they withdraw from their families and spend more time alone. David, for example, had begun to feel distant from his wife even before the drug use, but the Vicodin development in his life further isolated him—he was spending time alone driving to pharmacies all over his area and withdrawing by himself before popping his pills.

Confronting a Loved One Who Is Almost Addicted

So now that you know what to look for, suppose you conclude that a spouse or other loved one is almost addicted to drugs. Now what? How should you approach the individual? My first piece of advice is to not approach or confront the individual alone. Always try to have at least one other person present. These encounters can grow highly emotional. Another person can help provide a buffer and hopefully help prevent the conversation from descending into a shouting match or becoming too personal.

Although it can often be very difficult to maintain one's composure in the face of a loved one who is using drugs, it's best to stick to the facts and speak in as nonjudgmental a way as possible.

What you want to say are facts like "I found marijuana under the driver's seat of the car," "Your brother told me that you were acting erratically and appeared to have white powder around your nostrils," or similar factual statements. What you don't want to do is say "I think you have a problem with marijuana" or "I think you are abusing coke." Your loved one can much more easily deny or resist these harder-to-prove accusations.

Keep in mind that initially your loved one might be shocked when he's confronted if he genuinely thought that he'd been managing to conceal his drug use from everyone. I remember when a young man, age twenty-two, came to see me for his opiate addiction. He'd grown up in the same town outside of Boston where I live, and he knew that I lived there. He told me about a street in town where he and his friends used to go to buy, sell, and use drugs. I casually responded, "Oh, you mean

Washington Street?" and his jaw dropped. He had been convinced that only he and his friends knew about this drug hotspot and was shocked that an "outsider" like myself knew their "secret."

The same is often true for people who use drugs more generally—namely, they think nobody around them has a clue.

You should expect the person who is almost addicted—or anyone who uses drugs—to deny having a problem. Expect your loved one to question your sanity for even remotely suspecting drug use. Expect her to turn the tables and try to put you on the defensive for asking questions about drugs: "Are you crazy? Have I ever missed a family reunion? I have a job! I have two kids! Where would I even find drugs? When would I have *time* to use drugs?"

Again, it is the rare drug user who admits to using drugs at the first confrontation. Don't expect to immediately have a heart-to-heart conversation that gets to the bottom of it. Instead, it is more usual for the person to deny, conceal, and deflect any questions about drugs. As David's Vicodin habit progressed from almost addiction to addiction, once or twice people asked him if he was using and he, of course, denied any use whatsoever.

Once this initial confrontation has occurred, my advice is to insist that the individual be evaluated for substance use, preferably with a mental health worker who is knowledgeable about drug problems. Often this evaluation will include steps like urine drug screens or blood samples to determine whether the drug use is continuing or whether any medical problems have arisen as a result of the drug use.

The person may say he's only used once. Or that the drug use isn't a problem. Or that the mental health evaluation is a big waste of time and money. It doesn't matter. As you've already seen—and will continue to see throughout this book—even casual and occasional drug use can ruin someone's life (a physician or other professional can suffer a career-threatening incident even while using Vicodin that was obtained legitimately, like David did early in his almost addiction). Almost addiction is a genuine threat that requires definitive action.

What Families Can Do (and *Can't* Do) to Help a Loved One with Almost Addiction

One of the most important ways to help someone who is almost addicted actually comes off as the most important thing to *not* do: don't under any circumstance enable the person by covering up for his behavior or helping the drug use continue. Some of the advice above, as well as the questions that follow this section, is meant to root out enabling when it occurs and stop it.

The reason you don't want to enable drug use is that it not only allows the person who is using to continue her behavior without any significant change, but it also involves you compromising yourself in various ways, doing things that likely feel wrong on some level, and causing you to feel like less of a responsible human being than you want to be.

Also, since so much of another person's behavior is out of your control—and also because you may be too emotionally invested in the situation to make good choices yourself—insisting that your loved one start attending Alcoholics Anonymous (AA) or Narcotics Anonymous (NA) meetings is a good idea. "But I'm not an addict! I have nothing in common with these people! I have my life together!" Expect to hear responses like these, yet stick to your recommendation. Someone who is almost addicted does have something in common with the people in AA or NA. They all are using drugs (or have in the past), the drugs are causing problems already, the drugs could cause a life-changing catastrophe at any time, and the drug use could become worse.

Insist that the individual obtain a mental health evaluation. If reasonable and possible, ask that you be allowed both to offer information to assist the evaluation and to receive feedback from the evaluation so you can know exactly what the professional recommended.

No matter what course of action you choose, navigating these waters is almost always incredibly delicate, painful, and fraught with myriad unpleasant emotions.

As you're proceeding, remember that being almost addicted is unsafe, no matter how the user might try to convince himself —or you—otherwise. Any drug use can lead to dangerous outcomes in a multitude of ways. Almost addiction can and does create problems for the people who are using and for their families, even when it doesn't rise to the level of being a diagnosable substance abuse condition. Alone, almost addiction is a problem, even if it never grows worse. But remember, as in David's case, it can be a precursor to full-fledged addiction, replete with the accompanying destruction and devastation.

A Few Words on Home Drug Testing

Sometimes families will opt to drug test a family member themselves, using drug testing kits from the pharmacy to test the individual at random intervals or whenever they suspect drug use. Although there is some benefit of home drug testing,

I believe on the whole they are a waste of time, money, and emotional energy.

If a home drug test is positive, it provides clear evidence that your loved one is using drugs and that something should be done to decrease the chance that drug use will continue.

But often the test result will be negative, and these results can be falsely reassuring and, thus, dangerous. That's why I tend to discourage these tests. Let me explain. Suppose someone is using drugs but happens to be clean when a family member hands over a testing kit and insists on a urine sample. He can then point to the negative test result and say, "See—I told you I wasn't using! You were being unfair when you accused me, and I was telling the truth!" The person using drugs might actually be emboldened to keep using at the present level (or worse) given this drug test result, and the family members may be less likely to act on their concerns in the future.

Furthermore, there are many ways to "cheat" on a drug test. Be warned—this gets distasteful. Online outfits sell clean urine at low cost. People can easily substitute the stuff for their own unless someone actually observes them urinating into a cup. Also, if a test is not checking pH and creatinine levels, then it is possible to substitute water for urine or to heavily dilute a urine specimen that might otherwise be positive and obtain a clean result. Furthermore, some drugs of abuse are rarely screened for in home testing kits, including dextromethorphan, Salvia divinorum, and K2 (as well as its cousin Spice), a form of synthetic marijuana.

Drug testing for many elite athletes now mandates a "nipples to knees" policy for observing the collection of the urine specimen—the athletes must pull their clothing down to the knees and up to the chest while they're being observed urinating into a cup. Although this might seem like a draconian approach to the newcomer, it's for a reason. Guys can buy a battery-powered, strap-on attachment that expels urine and looks like the real appendage. Women can find crafty methods, as well. So without a nipples-to-knees policy, an observer can easily be fooled. Unless people actually watch a family member urinate, they cannot be completely confident that the person did not use substitute urine.

It's unlikely that many family members or loved ones would be eager to actually observe someone urinating into a cup to ensure the sample is not adulterated or substituted, especially if it's to address an almost addiction that hasn't caused serious personal or family problems yet.

So, all told, I think that although home drug testing can be valuable in a few situations, a negative test can be falsely reassuring and can cause the person using drugs to become even bolder in his patterns, thus putting himself into an even more dangerous situation.

Protect Yourself While Helping Your Loved One

Once you've come to the realization that your loved one may be almost addicted and then actually broached the topic with the person, you've started moving everyone toward a solution. As you proceed, it's important to keep yourself safe and healthy.

When someone in your home is using drugs, the chance increases that your medications will be stolen, your cash will disappear, and your jewelry will vanish, sometimes dramatically. As a result, you may need to take simple precautions, which often depend on the particular drug your loved one is using.

As you saw with David, some drugs pack more of an addictive potential than others, and some are much more expensive and harder to obtain. Opiates, as you saw in David's case, held such a pull for him that he couldn't avoid them. Being a doctor, his task of scoring drugs was relatively simple and didn't involve stealing from his family (aside from using his cousin's driver's license number). But in many cases, families get dragged along in the repercussions of a member's drug use, which can happen in both addiction and almost addiction.

Here are some things family members can do to help protect themselves.

Join a Self-Help Group
Al-Anon is without a doubt the biggest support group worldwide for families, loved ones, and other bystanders dealing with substance abuse. Many people attending the meetings are dealing with issues related to substances other than alcohol. Nar-Anon is another large, worldwide group available for concerned family members of people using drugs.

Joining these groups can provide you with useful information on navigating the repercussions of a loved one's almost addiction. Participating will also confirm that you are not alone—plus, it sends a message to your loved one that you're taking the problem seriously.

Reach Out
Talk to others in your family or close friends. Talking about what you're facing will remind you that you are not alone, and other people (who may have dealt with similar problems) may offer solutions that you hadn't considered.

Seek Professional Help

I have worked with many concerned family members who came in—sometimes with their loved one who was using drugs and sometimes alone—seeking counsel and advice about how to proceed. Sometimes the question is simply "Do you think I'm missing a substance abuse problem?" Other times the person in my office is certain about the drug abuse and wants advice on how to respond. Sometimes people have a plan but fear they're being too strict and harsh (or, more rarely, too lenient) in implementing the plan.

Do Not Allow Yourself to Be Abused

In the midst of drug use, including almost addiction, spouses and families can face abuse in all forms—emotional, physical, financial, and occasionally sexual. You aren't required to be a punching bag, nor should you be one.

If your loved one is stealing from you, consider reporting it to the authorities. Failing to do so might be enabling the loved one and simply reinforcing her problem. You shouldn't ever tolerate physical abuse. If someone's good judgment has been set aside for the influence of an intoxicating substance, the stage is set for physical abuse.

My strong advice is that if any physical abuse occurs, you should report it immediately and make every effort to stop it. I have seen too many people in therapy who have suffered abuse that went unchecked or unreported, and they wonder aloud why nobody tried to stop it by calling the police or seeking help otherwise. The experience leaves them questioning their own worth. On the other hand, many of my patients over the years who were almost addicted or truly addicted have had family members call 911 when they became physically abusive.

Emotional abuse is often more difficult to label and sometimes harder to know how to handle. That's because the event isn't necessarily as clear cut as being physically struck or being robbed of family heirlooms. Regardless, once it is clear that emotional abuse is occurring, family members should try to remove themselves from hurtful situations as much as possible.

Focus on Your Own Health and Well-Being

Eating right, getting enough sleep, exercising, and keeping up your doctor's appointments helps you to concentrate your efforts and attention on something for which you have a direct say on the outcome—yourself. Making sure that you have time to go to the gym or for a walk isn't selfish; it's sensible.

On a similar note, avoid turning to alcohol or illicit drugs in order to endure the pain or to cope. These kinds of activities not only harm you; they also make it less likely that you'll be able to help initiate and maintain the changes that your loved one needs. Plus, it doesn't set a good example at the very time your loved one needs it.

Avoid Being Part of the Cover-Up

Although perfect strangers don't need to know your family's business, those in your inner circle, mental health professionals and doctors you might visit, clergy, and others close to you should know about what's transpiring at home. All of these people can join any efforts you're trying, and they can help you reach your goals. They may also be able to reach out to your almost addicted loved one themselves, helping to reinforce the message you're sending.

Educate Yourself about Substance Abuse and Addiction

In the adolescent substance abuse program where I work at Children's Hospital Boston, we have various ways of educating families about drug use. We offer guidance sessions to parents whose kids are using drugs. We also offer support group meetings for parents, which are facilitated by one of the social workers in the program.

These groups not only show parents that they are not alone in their travails, but also serve as powerful approaches for educating them about all aspects of drug use, including how to set limits for their children and watch for observations that serve as warning signs. Every few months a physician in the program will attend these nighttime groups and offer scientific information about the physiological and biochemical effects of drug use. We offer these talks because we feel that every bit of added information provides support and assistance for family members struggling with a loved one's drug use.

David's Outcome

After his arrest, the police assumed that David must be selling Vicodin because they thought, incorrectly, that no one could be taking as much as he was and not have anyone around him know about it, much less be able to function as a doctor.

David cooperated fully with the police and FBI investigations of his drug use (the FBI was involved because some of the pharmacies he used were in a bordering state), and they eventually concluded that David was indeed providing only himself with an extremely high dose of pills. He eventually entered a plea agreement, avoided jail time, and finished his year of probation without incident.

He'd begun recovering his sobriety; then came the grueling task of recovering his job. As soon as he was discharged from the treatment facility, David entered a chemical dependency monitoring contract with the state physician health program. This required regular meetings with a psychiatrist, attending AA meetings, and submitting to random urine drug screens.

After two and a half years of remaining clean, along with carefully negotiating with the state's board of registration in medicine, David returned to psychiatric practice. Between being out of work and attending therapy after his arrest, David had a lot of time to think about what kind of psychiatric work he might like to do, so when he returned he took a moderate pay cut from his previous salary and entered a practice at three-fourths time (75 percent of full time) in which he had full control over his schedule and could see patients for whatever length of time he wished. His pay directly reflected how many patients he saw—compared to his previous job where his pay was fixed regardless of how many patients he saw—and he never felt better.

I continued to work with David for six years after he returned to practice and he remained clean, sober, and content in his work. However, his marriage continued to suffer, and eventually he divorced, but I don't think his drug use factored into the divorce.

Even though his story continued happily, or relatively so, David didn't have to lose himself in the frenzied business of chasing down Vicodin all over the city in the first place. He didn't have to get arrested. He didn't have to lose his license and his ability to practice medicine in order to get his drug use straightened out. If his intervention had occurred earlier, his almost addiction could have been nipped with much less pain before it became a full-fledged addiction.

■ ◆ ■

| 7 |

Unsafe at Any Age
Almost Addicted Across the Life Span

No matter when it occurs, almost addiction is a dangerous development for people young, old, and in between.

Because of the way their brains are developing, adolescents are at particular risk of becoming almost addicted, and they're at higher risk of negative outcomes from drug use.

Older people, on the other hand, may be more likely to become almost addicted because they may have more time on their hands, fewer people monitoring their behavior, and greater access to prescription drugs. But the impact of taking unnecessary drugs can hit seniors especially hard, since they're more likely to have health problems that are worsened by drug use.

A young man named Nick who turned up in my office can provide lessons for both young and older people who are almost addicted.

Nick's Story

Nick was eighteen years old when he wound up in our emergency department. He had gotten drunk at a party, where he proclaimed that he was going to kill himself. He was yelling this repeatedly and becoming more and more belligerent when a former girlfriend called 911 and police came and brought him to our facility. He told emergency workers that he had a number of immediate stressors in his life, including his lack of a job and a strained relationship with the ex-girlfriend.

When I first met him, Nick said he smoked marijuana about once a month, but had used it more frequently several years earlier. He also said he used Klonopin—a prescription drug used to relieve panic attacks—on occasion.

From birth, Nick's life had been painful and stressful. He was raised in public housing. His parents frequently fought, both verbally and physically, until his father moved out when Nick was five. He witnessed fights almost daily in the projects, often with bloodshed. Although his father had moved to a neighboring town, Nick never saw him. He and his five siblings were raised by his mother in their apartment.

Nick recalled that he'd had trouble controlling his behavior since he was young. He also said he had a long history of stealing, which dated back to elementary school, and he would break into cars for fun. Behaviors like these led him to be diagnosed with ADHD in elementary school, but the treatment didn't do much to help.

Despite the problems he experienced earlier in life, almost the first event that Nick told me about was a biking accident at age eleven. He and his best friend were horsing around, jumping curbs and dodging potholes on their bikes. He remembered seeing the flash of a car to his right, seemingly out of nowhere, and nothing after that. The car hit both boys, killing the friend instantly and leaving Nick in a coma for four weeks.

Afterward, he began the slow process of physical rehabilitation. He was devastated over his friend's death and years later still thought of him almost every day. When I met him, he said he was filled with sadness over this death, two of his friends' recent suicides, and the death of an uncle.

Despite his sadness and traumatic brain injury, Nick didn't think his behavior changed much after the accident. He continued to have problems paying attention and getting into trouble in school, just as he had before the injury. He'd been in psychiatric treatment off and on after the bike accident, but hadn't seen anyone consistently for years. Since being diagnosed with ADHD as a child, he'd been prescribed various medications over the years but never took anything steadily enough to help much.

Several years before I met Nick, he tried to kill himself. He said he was home alone, thinking again about his friend's death, and decided he had nothing to live for. He called his brother just after he swallowed an entire bottle of Tylenol and told him what he'd done. His brother called 911 and emergency personnel arrived within minutes, transporting him to a nearby emergency room, where staffers pumped his stomach and admitted him to a psychiatric unit for treatment.

Mental illness and drug use were common among his family members, including a brother with marijuana dependence, a sister with depression, and several family members with likely post-traumatic stress disorder.

The Dangers of Being Almost Addicted in Adolescence

Problems with drugs often start during people's teen years. One large-scale study concluded that approximately 15 percent of all adults will eventually develop a substance use problem of some sort and that the median age of onset of the substance use disorder was twenty.[63]

Thus, for many individuals, substance use begins in adolescence. Indeed, many adolescents seem to be inviting almost addiction into their lives these days. During 2010, 25 percent of eighth, tenth, and twelfth graders in the United States reported using marijuana in the previous year. This same survey found that 17 percent of high school seniors had abused illicit drugs other than marijuana during the past year, including drugs such as the stimulants Ritalin and Adderall, tranquilizers such as Xanax, and opiate painkillers such as OxyContin and Vicodin. More seniors had abused tranquilizers or prescription narcotics in the past year than heroin and cocaine combined.[64]

Although someone might begin to use drugs for many reasons—including psychological, genetic, and cultural reasons—the influence of one's peers is probably the single greatest factor during the teen and post-teen years. Many teens and young adults feel a great deal of pressure to fit in with their friends and acquaintances.

The age at which young people start using drugs heavily influences the extent to which drugs will play a part in their lives. Research has shown that the younger people are when they first use drugs, the higher their chance of eventually becoming addicted after age eighteen.[65] Therefore, even a single episode of drug use at a young age can be like rolling the dice to determine where the individual will end up. Because of this, identifying and intervening in almost addicted behaviors among adolescents and young adults may be even more important than doing so for older adults.

Various physiological factors can explain why adolescents are so vulnerable. Because the physical size of a person's brain reaches its peak between the ages of ten and twenty, experts long thought that brain development stopped around ages twelve to fourteen. However, neuroscience now believes that the brain continues to develop until the early twenties. Because the brain is maturing throughout adolescence, a teenager's brain is exquisitely sensitive to any environmental input or insult. As such, drug use at this stage of life is particularly problematic.[66]

What exactly are some of the brain changes that occur during adolescence? First of all, brain development occurs in waves and stages, and the evolutionarily older, more primitive parts of the brain develop first.[67] These more basic regions are the parts that oversee reward seeking and pleasurable activities. As such, these areas of the brain relish stimulation and excitement and are the areas most affected by illicit drug use.

However, the higher-order parts of the brain are those that govern rational thinking, setting limits, impulse control, and judgment. These decide whether one should act on those deeper impulses that arise from more primitive areas of the brain. Unfortunately, these regions develop later and more slowly than the reward-seeking portions.

The end result of this developmental mismatch can lead to scary moments that are familiar to most people who've been around adolescents. The thrill-seeking part of the brain develops earlier in life than the part of the brain that is logical and rational and that considers the consequences of behaviors. This helps explain why adolescents are more likely to engage in impulsive, risky behaviors such as experimenting with drugs. At the same time the reward system has kicked into high gear and kids are most vulnerable to the pleasurable effects of drugs, their cognitive capacity to evaluate risk and benefits and think about the long-term effects of any decision is still evolving.

This discrepancy—and the resulting vulnerability to drugs—is compounded if the young person has a genetic predisposition toward drug abuse, if drugs and drug use are common in his environment, or if he is suffering from emotional distress or has ADHD.[68]

Studies have repeatedly shown that teens respond differently to drugs than adults do. One particularly important difference is that young people tend to be less sensitive to the adverse effects of substances of abuse. As a result, teens are less likely to become sedated by tranquilizing drugs like benzodiazepines, and instead are more likely to remain alert and awake while under the influence. Because of this, teens may be able to stay awake longer while intoxicated, which in turn can allow them to take even more of the drug. Where an adult might fall asleep before getting behind the wheel or logging on to the computer or heading to another party, a teen may be more likely to remain awake and start driving, chatting online with strangers, or making all manner of other potentially life-changing decisions.

When adolescents use marijuana, the white matter of their brains can undergo changes that are similar to what occurs in the brains of individuals with schizophrenia.[69] Perhaps it's not surprising, then, that marijuana smoking in adolescence significantly increases the risk for later schizophrenia. The risk is even greater for people who had psychiatric symptoms before their first experience with marijuana and those with schizophrenia in their families. Young people who use marijuana are also at increased risk for developing anxiety and depression, which in turn can foster the desire to use drugs more heavily.[70]

Also, adolescents with a substance use disorder are known to attempt suicide and successfully kill themselves more frequently than adolescents without a substance use disorder, and if these adolescents also have depression, they are much more likely to commit suicide.

Separately, having ADHD—as Nick did—makes people more likely to develop a problem with substance abuse. Surveys found that 9.5 percent of US youths ages four to seventeen had been diagnosed with ADHD in 2007.[71] This condition is by no means limited to the United States. Research from 2007 that looked at 102 earlier studies involving more than 171,000 people from around the world found that about 5.3 percent of people worldwide have ADHD. Rates appeared to be similar in North America and Europe.[72]

What Parents and Other Concerned Adults Can Do

As you can see, teenagers are at special risk of developing almost addiction for many reasons. And the consequences of their drug use can be both immediate and long ranging. If you're reading this book because you're concerned about a teen's possible drug use, it's important to realize that adults can do a lot to help adolescents in these situations.

Become Aware of the Problem

The first goal is to recognize that the substance use is occurring. Doing so can be difficult, because teens are remarkably good at covering their tracks. Most teens know that any use is likely to draw the attention of authorities or other adults, so they usually try to hide every aspect of their drug use. Unfortunately teens often spend a lot of time sequestered away in their rooms, they can come into contact with many kids at school who have access to drugs, and they can stay in constant communication with their peer network through cell phones and computers—all of which are tools that can foster an almost addiction.

Over the years, I have seen parents who had absolutely no knowledge or suspicion of drug use until the teen let his guard down just enough to allow the parents a rare peek into his life. For one mother, her son just looked bleary-eyed. Another parent smelled marijuana on her child. Another mom's suspicion was raised only after she inadvertently stumbled upon her son's instant messaging on his computer. Yet another only investigated after the mother of her child's friend called to say she'd discovered that her own kid was using drugs.

Because of my experience with adolescents, my advice to parents and family members is that if they have any suspicion of drug use, they ought to explore their concerns and not try to sweep them under the rug or explain them away. If you have evidence that your child or teen has used illicit drugs even once, that's reason enough to launch a full investigation and develop a plan to prevent drug use from occurring a second time.

I'm reminded of one of my elderly patients who had three grown children, including a daughter who had experienced drug problems years earlier as an adolescent. My patient said she had no idea whatsoever that her daughter was using drugs until she and her husband were out with another couple. My patient and the other woman got up from the dinner table to go to the ladies' room together, and as they entered the restroom, my patient sniffed a couple of times and said, "Someone else is wearing my daughter's perfume." Her friend turned toward her and responded with surprise, "That's not perfume. That's marijuana!"

Although this anecdote may be amusing, overlooking adolescents' drug use that "merely" rises to the level of almost addiction can allow them to move toward very *un*funny consequences.

If you're a parent or other caregiver, it's important to remain vigilant and proactive about drug use in teens. If you're not sure what to make of clues you're gathering, I recommend conferring with a health care professional or other parents who might have experienced something similar before you reach a conclusion.

Get the Teen's Attention

If you do strongly suspect or have direct knowledge that your child is using drugs, what steps should you take? In a word, it's all about *leverage:* How much leverage do you have over the young person? What rewards or privileges do you control that the teen wants, hopefully badly, and that you can use as a bargaining tool to guide her into different behavior? One of the keys for utilizing this kind of leverage is finding just the right factor to use. You can't deprive young people of something essential for life or well-being—like food or shelter—but you can't hope to succeed by using a nicety that they don't really care about either.

In the adolescent substance abuse program in which I work, we have formulated "The Seven Cs" as a shorthand reminder of various tools for applying leverage over young people; they are cash, car, computer, curfew, cell phone, and credit cards ("credit cards" counts for two Cs). My advice to parents whose child is already engaged in problematic drug use (and in most instances any use is problematic) is to limit the child's access to some or all of the Seven Cs. Not only are the Seven Cs vital for maintaining a teen's social network and hunger for entertainment, but they also play important roles in an adolescent's ability to obtain more drugs.

Because life is rarely black and white, there are times when the line between what is essential for the child and what is optional becomes blurred. For example, many homework assignments require access to a computer and the Internet, so completely banning the computer is simply not feasible for many teens if you want them to succeed in school. Nor should you keep a student from carrying cash that is needed to buy lunch. But short of an absolute need for one of these Cs, you can leverage all of these items as tools for limiting access to drug use or to provide rewards or encouragement for good choices.

Take the Drug Use Seriously—Even If It's Hard to Accept That It's Happening

Even when parents are aware of drug use, their will to take action often comes up short. Parents and other concerned adults may convince themselves that a teenager just can't get by without a computer or absolutely needs cash on hand or a credit card at all times for emergencies.

The Seven Cs of Leverage

All of these elements of teens' lives play a big role in their happiness . . . and their ability to obtain drugs. By limiting or restricting any or all of these privileges, you can motivate adolescents who are almost addicted to want to change their behavior, plus make it harder to get drugs even if they still want to use. If it's not practical to make an outright ban on one of these Cs, here's how to supervise how your teen uses it:

- **Cash.** If you dole out the cash, provide only enough for necessities, and ask for an accounting of how it's spent. If the teen has a job, know how much he's bringing in and ask for a general explanation of where it goes.

- **Credit cards.** Be sure to check their statements each month.

- **Computer.** If she must have access, track your teen's computer usage by checking the computer's history, reviewing her social-networking usage, and installing software to keep tabs on how the computer has been used.

- **Curfew.** Be sure to stay awake until your teen has arrived home, and try to stay aware of any unapproved excursions in the night.

- **Cell phone.** If the teen must have a phone, ask to review the phone bill at the end of the month so you can see who she's calling and texting.

- **Car.** Be sure the odometer matches up with the amount of driving your teen is allowed to do.

Other parents will ignore signs of concern or take a teen's denials at face value, turn a blind eye, and hope for the best. Still others may simply be too busy to deal with anything but an emergency, and a child whose good grades and after-school activities conceal an almost addiction may not set off any warning bells.

Another reason that parents might hesitate to prevent further drug use is that they themselves used a little cocaine or smoked some weed when they were younger. As a result, some parents will assure themselves that drug use is a normal phase of development that their kids will eventually outgrow. But here's a reality check: the marijuana sold today is ten to fifty times stronger than that sold three decades ago. Plus, most parents want to give their kids every opportunity for success and keep away all the elements that will hold them back or knock them off track. Even just a little drug use at this point in their lives can reduce their potential for success.

Other parents who *still* use drugs from time to time may feel hypocritical insisting that their child stay clean. If you take drugs occasionally and don't feel they cause problems in your life, perhaps the concern that you're modeling inappropriate behavior might be a sign that it's time for you to stop, too.

Still other parents may have never enforced appropriate limits or boundaries even when their kids were young, and they feel incapable of beginning now with substance misuse during the teen years.

Given that teenagers can be crafty in sneaking drugs and alcohol, as well as relentless in their badgering and hectoring, I definitely concede that enforcing limits on uncooperative offspring can be exhausting. But the stakes are too high at this critical time of development to ponder the alternative.

Clearly State Your Expectations about Drug Use

This might sound obvious, but you should be talking to your kids regularly about general issues in their lives. And regarding drug use in particular, it is important to explicitly state that you do not want them to use drugs. Studies show that kids whose parents talk to them about drugs, set clear rules about drug use, and also follow through with consequences for breaking those rules use fewer drugs than kids whose parents don't do so. A recent British study found that adolescents whose parents discouraged them from drinking alcohol used relatively few mind-altering substances.[73]

Know Where Your Kids Are

Setting expectations about your teens' whereabouts is an important way to show them that you care about their safety and well-being. It's also important that you be willing to intervene should they go someplace that is unsafe, plan to be with someone who is dangerous in some way, or fail to return home when expected. Although doing these things is no guarantee that any child will remain drug-free, teens who know they are loved, cared for, and respected will fare better on average than those who don't—even if they protest.

Talk to Their Friends' Parents

Other parents are potentially valuable sources of information; they may have heard what your teen is doing (or not doing) and which kids might be using drugs and which ones are likely not. Conversing regularly with other parents can provide an illuminating perspective on what's happening when your teen is away from home.

Plan More Face Time with Your Teen

Spend plenty of time around your adolescent. Doing so gives parents an invaluable look into their kids' day-to-day lives. What kind of music do they listen to? What inspires them? Who do they look up to? Go jogging or biking with them on the weekends. Incorporate them into your hobbies, and ask if they'll share theirs with you.

And eat meals together whenever possible. One study found that teens who ate dinner with their families fewer than three times per week were three and a half times more likely to have abused prescription drugs, three times more likely to have used marijuana, and 50 percent more likely to have used alcohol than teens who ate dinner with their families five or more times per week.[74]

Act Swiftly on Your Hunches

Don't waste any time if you think your child is using drugs or even just hanging out with kids who are. Because experimentation or occasional drug use can quickly morph into problematic use, abuse, or addiction, acting quickly and decisively to limit a child's exposure to illicit drugs is vital. If you suspect use, seek professional help and insist on an evaluation. If your teen refuses to participate, employ whatever leverage you can to ensure cooperation.

Stay Savvy about Technology

Many adolescents get information about drugs from the Internet, and many use some form of messaging—either on their computers, their cell phones, or both—to obtain drugs. Although teens need privacy, if your teen's behavior online or with a cell phone changes dramatically (for example, she becomes more secretive or begins to keep her phone always on her person), then don't rule out the possibility that drugs are somehow involved. Hopefully a new (drug-free) love interest has caused the cell phone to become even more of a body appendage than it already was, but without further information, you are right to suspect that the change could be linked to drug use.

A Cautionary Tale from My Own Experience

Although I've certainly seen my share of teen drug and alcohol use in my psychiatric work, I have also unfortunately seen firsthand the ways that teens can outwit even the best-laid parental plans.

A couple of years ago, my wife—who is also a Harvard physician—and I hosted an all-night high school graduation party for one of our daughters, who was graduating from boarding school in New Hampshire. A friend had graciously offered that we could stay in his home, which was near the campus, and host a graduation party there. The house had plenty of lawn space to pitch tents, and our plan was to serve pizza and soft drinks for dinner and a simple breakfast the next morning before the teens headed out.

My daughter invited her whole class—roughly 125 students —to the party and, in two separate emails beforehand, declared that it was a no-alcohol, no-drug event. Probably two-thirds of the class actually came to the party. Once it got under way and we were about to serve the pizza, my wife and I stood on a picnic table on the lawn, gathered all the kids, and both stated there was to be no alcohol and no drugs, and then asked if everyone present agreed to abide by these rules. Everyone nodded assent. At that moment, I felt happy to be able to host a party for all the new graduates. Little did I know that roughly four hours later things would drastically change.

A couple hours later, things were moving along without any apparent problems. My wife and I and another parent couple mingled with the kids and saw nothing improper. Around 9 p.m. I told the other couple that everything looked fine and they left, planning to return early in the morning to begin cooking breakfast. My wife and I continued to wander through the party, which was both inside and outside the house, and saw nothing of concern except one kid playing a boom box a bit too loudly. Twice we had to ask him to turn it down.

Neighbors apparently heard the music as well, because at least one of them called the police to complain about noise. At about 11 p.m., I was playing Ping-Pong with a couple of the boys on the first floor when I noticed a flashlight shining in the window. I walked outside to investigate and saw a police officer. I said hello and he asked, "Is this your party?" When I said it was, he told me I was under arrest for "hosting an underage drinking party," spun me around, cuffed me, and put me in the back of his cruiser. Before arresting me, they'd caught several kids outside consuming alcohol.

They also arrested my wife a short time later and brought both of us—along with seventy or so kids—to the local station. The kids were released after several hours to their parents or another adult. While we were there, the police showed us photographs they'd taken of the house and property, and we were astonished to see beer cans in various places inside the house as well as strewn on the lawn and inside tents. The police told us that they found cases of beer in several kids' car trunks. We were held until morning, charged with criminal mis-demeanors, and then released on bail.

How had we missed all of that alcohol? One of the kids later told us that they knew when we were walking through and simply hid the can or glass and kept it out of our sight until we passed by.

Soon after we got home, the press descended upon us. We thought about simply saying "No comment," but we decided that offering that response might make it appear like we either supplied the alcohol or, at a minimum, condoned it. So against our lawyers' advice, I spoke to each television crew that arrived as well as with every newspaper reporter who called. Ultimately the criminal charges were dropped, but the damage was done.

Looking back, as my wife and I have done countless times, we were incredibly naive about hosting such a large party for teenagers. As she's said, once we agreed to host the party, the rest was almost a fait accompli. Maybe if we had several dozen chaperones along with police present from the outset, things would've gone better, but even in situations that have those safeguards in place I've heard of kids consuming alcohol and drugs anyway. (Since my arrest, I've heard every possible permutation of graduation party horror stories.) As embarrassing and painful as our arrests have been, we're lucky that the police broke up the party when they did, because given how much alcohol we saw in their photographs, some kids might have been harmed had they continued to drink throughout the night.

I'm telling this story to make quite clear that I'm not talking about teen substance use merely from a clinical perspective, but also as someone who's been there and been burned. Perhaps my story can help you see substance use among adolescents a little more clearly and take appropriate action when necessary.

Substance Abuse at the Other End of the Age Spectrum

Almost addicted behavior at any age is concerning, and adolescence may be the most dangerous period for such drug use, but almost addiction among seniors may run a close second in terms of the danger of negative consequences. Some might assume that older adults would never engage in illicit drug use, or at least that if they were to use drugs, they wouldn't do so at harmful levels. After all, older people have accumulated enough wisdom in life to tell the bad ideas from the good ones, right? And wouldn't their need for quick thrills fade decades after their adolescence and young adult years?

At any rate, some bystanders might assume that since getting older comes with so many health problems in itself that once you are old, any drug use you get into couldn't be more harmful than normal aging.

All of those assumptions are wrong.

First of all, many older people do use illicit drugs. Substance use among older adults has risen sharply. One national survey in the United States, for example, found that between 2002 and 2007, roughly 49 percent of individuals ages fifty to fifty-nine had used illicit substances at some point during their lives.[75]

This demographic is the same cohort of folks who saw drug use as practically normal behavior from the late 1960s through the early 1980s, so it's not surprising that so many adults in this age range have used drugs at some point in their lives. But plenty were still using drugs more recently; 5 percent of adults ages fifty-five to fifty-nine had used illicit drugs in the previous month in 2008.[76]

So, older people are using plenty of drugs. And when they do so, they face dangers that are different from those that young people encounter—but just as real. Any drug use among older individuals is potentially much more dangerous than for younger adults. The normal aging process involves the loss of brain cells, a decrease in general organ function, and greater susceptibility to infections, and therefore more vulnerability to any drug of abuse. Not only do the organs that clear drugs from your system (primarily the kidneys and liver) usually work more slowly than earlier in life, but the brain tissue of older adults is more vulnerable to damage from any drug of abuse.

Thus, older individuals are at much higher risk for dangerous levels of intoxication from drugs compared to other adults, even when they use them minimally. The same amount of any drug will likely hit an older individual much harder than it will affect someone who is younger.

This fact is well known in medical circles and applies to therapeutic medications as well, hence the adage when prescribing medicines for older folks: start low and go slow.

Aging also brings a number of complicating factors that put older adults at higher risk of almost addiction. First, they tend to experience more pain—arthritis becomes more common with age, for example—and many are prescribed opiate pain medications for their conditions. Physicians might assume that because patients are older, they may be at less risk of abusing these medications. Conversely, for their part, patients might assume that because a drug is prescribed by a doctor, it can't be bad for them. They then let their guard down about misusing the drug and take more than they should or use it in other inappropriate ways.

Statistics clearly show that some people who are prescribed opiate pain medications develop substance use disorders as a result. Patients in pain who also have either depression or anxiety (as is the case for many older adults) are at even greater risk for problematic use of opiate medications.

To compound the danger, the number of prescription medications that the average older adult is taking can be staggering. One US study found that 44 percent of men ages sixty-five or older use five or more medications per week, and 12 percent use ten or more each week; among older women, those figures were 57 percent and 12 percent.[77] And a Swedish study found that among adults ages sixty-five and older, women used an average of 4.8 prescription medications and men used an average of 3.8.[78]

Among older adults, whose balance or reflexes might already be waning, even modest illicit drug use can increase the likelihood of falling, motor vehicle accidents, or other forms of trauma. These can result in broken bones, brain bleeding, and other severe injuries that may require a long convalescence—if they can even be overcome.

What Family Members and Concerned Others Should Look For

Despite the dangers, almost addiction among older adults can easily be overlooked. For starters, older people may not get out of the house as often as younger people do, and they may not have to show up anywhere such as a workplace on a regular basis. As such, they are often scrutinized much less closely than younger adults who are expected to come to work, drop kids off at school, and juggle countless household chores. Second, becoming a little slower mentally is commonplace in older folks, and many symptoms of drug use can resemble the symptoms that may occur with age in general.

When watching for the signs of almost addiction in older people, keep an eye out for the following red flags:

Forgetfulness or Rapid Cognitive Decline
These serve as two of the most basic signs of almost addiction in older people. However, the initial decline might be very hard to notice.

For example, one older man who has been my patient for many years had been quite sociable and intelligent. But even though I saw him regularly, I didn't pick up the extent to which his mental faculties had declined until I asked him to draw a clock face, complete with numbers and hands, that showed four o'clock.

Despite his impressive verbal abilities, most of the twelve numbers were on the left side of the clock, and although the long hand pointed due north (as it should), the short hand pointed due south, toward where the six should be. Once we established that he could draw a clock correctly just a few years earlier, it was hard to say exactly what had contributed to his declining mental faculties. Was the alcohol he'd heavily abused two decades earlier finally catching up to him? Was the decline due to normal aging? Dementia? Overuse of his prescription opiate painkillers?

Frequent Falling
Even though falling, with subsequent bone fractures, is common among the elderly, a sudden increase in falls or other mishaps that result in physical harm may point to possible drug use.

I work with several older individuals whose accidents have dramatically increased in frequency as they've aged. In one of them, I suspect that heavy alcohol use contributed to the problem, and in another patient I suspect that misuse of opiate pain medications is partly to blame.

Other behaviors that might indicate problematic drug use among older adults include

- spending more and more time alone
- asking to not be visited
- behaving in a more secretive or paranoid manner

Any or all of these behaviors could indicate drug use, but they could also suggest some type of brain damage, depression, anxiety, or another mental health problem.

Warning Signs of Almost Addiction in Older Adults

These signs don't automatically point to drug misuse in older adults, since some can occur simply with age. But if these crop up in an older friend or loved one, it's worth investigating whether inappropriate drug use may be contributing or whether the individual has a health problem that needs to be addressed:

- More forgetfulness
- Lots of time alone
- Secrecy or paranoia
- Rapid cognitive decline
- Frequent falling
- Nodding off or sleeping at odd times

What You Can Do

So what can be done once a substance use problem is discovered in someone who is older? The answer depends in part on the nature and type of problem. In some ways, the simplest drug problem to address in older adults is the kind that seems to have arisen through confusion or misunderstanding about how to take pills properly. Such problems can often be solved simply by having a family member or a visiting nurse place the proper medications into a pill box or just dispense the medications directly to the individual rather than letting him keep the full bottle.

The situation becomes murkier when an older individual who is almost addicted pretends to not understand how to take the medications when in reality she knows that she is taking too much. In these instances, one should talk to the person, while airing concerns about misuse, and take measures to limit access to the drugs. The older person's physician may need to be included in finding a solution.

The problem is probably most difficult to address in people who have their full cognitive capacities and have been abusing substances throughout their adult life and, as they get older, are simply continuing their use as before. Until something happens that dramatically throws their problematic use into focus—like a DUI, a breakup in which the significant other cites substance use as the culprit, or a positive drug test—getting them to change their behavior late in life is difficult.

However, change is always possible, and it can come for unclear or unknown reasons. In one hospital where I used to admit patients to a detox facility, the most well-known patient on the detox ward had more than 150 admissions over a fifteen-year period. His multivolume medical record occupied nearly ten feet in the medical records room (in today's electronic records, it would take up a good chunk of a hard drive). But one day he simply stopped using. Hospital workers would occasionally see him around town and uniformly comment on how good—and sober—he looked, and nobody knew why he stopped.

If you're concerned about an older loved one who may be almost addicted, making this point may be helpful in spurring change: Getting old *is* often hard. People lose their mental sharpness and physical fitness. They make more and more trips to the doctor's office to limit the effects of diseases. When you consider all the work it takes to feel good in your later years, why deliberately do something that counteracts all that effort, even just occasionally? Illicit drugs—whether it's pot or cocaine or prescriptions that are misused—aren't going to help. Instead, they just leave people less able to deal with the challenges of older age.

Advice to Share with an Older Person Who Is Almost Addicted

If an older loved one's drug use has pushed her into almost addiction, try these recommendations:

Ask Why the Drug Use Is Occurring

It's important for you to understand what factors may be fueling your loved one's drug use. Ask the following questions:

- Are you taking drugs because you are lonely? Bored?
- Do you feel like the meaning for your life ended when you stopped working?
- Are you feeling down and depressed and aren't sure exactly why?

These are common feelings among older adults, but there are far better ways of dealing with them than taking illicit drugs. Suggest that your loved one visit a doctor or mental health professional, and volunteer to come along for the visit.

Ask for a Medication Review

Ask your loved one's primary care doctor to review all the medications she's taking. Because older individuals often take many different prescription medications, it is all too easy for them to become confused about what to take. This can lead to inadvertent drug abuse. Taking multiple medications also increases the chance that someone might become confused as a side effect of their prescriptions, which in turn can lead to inadvertent problematic use.

I see one gentleman in his seventies who is prescribed a total of twelve medications for everything from shingles pain to depression to high blood pressure. Although he tries to take his medications as directed, he has wound up in emergency rooms roughly half a dozen times in the past decade for falling, becoming lethargic, or acting confused, just from inadvertently taking his medications incorrectly.

Because polypharmacy (being prescribed numerous medications at the same time) is so common among older patients, their doctors should review their medication list regularly and stop any drugs whose need is unclear. Ask the doctor to consider whether any ongoing medications have the potential for addiction and, if so, how to deal with this concern. Once they are discontinued, any unused pills should be disposed of properly to eliminate the chance that the person will take or abuse an old medication at some later time.

Encourage Social Activities

Isolation is dangerous for older folks. If an older person starts to draw inward, the connection with the outside world—along with the need to be accountable to others—diminishes. This can set the stage for unusual or dangerous behaviors, including almost addiction, that go unchecked. Involve your older loved one in family activities and social outings. Visit his home regularly to keep tabs on his behavior. Urge him to join social groups in his area or to volunteer with organizations that interest him.

Encourage Physical Activity

Remaining physically active often staves off many of the more debilitating and troublesome aspects of aging. Exercise can preserve muscle mass, bone strength, and mental clarity, among other benefits. If the physical activity is done in the company of others—thereby increasing one's social contact—all the better.

Encourage your loved one to join a gym, sign up for an aerobics program, or take part in a walking group.

Nick's Outcome

Nick's brain trauma and coma undoubtedly left him more vulnerable to the damaging, intoxicating effects of drugs than he would have been otherwise. To compound the problem, Nick hadn't been facing his challenges before his accident from a position of strength, either. He experienced his share of trauma growing up, which itself hits the brain hard, and he also had to deal with ADHD.

After discussing how vulnerable his brain was and how sensitive it likely would be to any prescription we might begin, we agreed that it was nonetheless in Nick's best interest to start taking stimulant medication for his impulsivity and ADHD. I am hesitant to prescribe stimulants for anyone, much less individuals who have any history of criminal activity or illicit substance use—because stimulants are valuable on the street and are frequently misused. Nonetheless, there was a sincerity and vulnerability surrounding Nick that made me want to believe that he intended to do more with his life.

Although I believe that treatment with the medication helped, it was only one of several steps that Nick was taking to get away from his previous life—and the friends who used drugs or committed crimes. He began staying at an aunt's house several towns away, got a job in a local supermarket with room for advancement, and stopped using all drugs.

I also feel strongly that having a supportive, nonjudgmental, and nurturing relationship within the context of our visits was also helpful. If you suspect that a loved one of any age is sliding into almost addiction, you can be that caring person and provide the help to begin turning away from drugs.

❖

Part 4

Solutions for Your Almost Addiction

Author's Note

In the previous chapters I've been addressing two groups: people concerned about their own drug use and people concerned about a loved one's drug use. It's often a friend or family member who first recognizes the problem and seeks help. Part 4 speaks directly to people using drugs who are seeking help on their own or who were handed this book by a loved one and now believe their drug use may be a problem—that they might be almost addicted.

8

Time for a Change
Helping Yourself

Many people who decide to live a drug-free life find that doing so isn't easy.

Like the people featured in this book, you may have found that using marijuana, hallucinogens, cocaine, speed, or Vicodin adds something to your life that you're missing. Perhaps a drug perks you up, relaxes you, or gives you a lens for looking at the world that makes it more appealing. Clearly, you have found *some* reason to use a drug, and turning away from it will require effort, as you learn how to live without the benefit you perceive from it.

In addition, drug use may be woven into your daily routine by now. Obtaining and using it may occupy a set time in your schedule. It may give you something to do with friends and acquaintances. For some people who are almost addicted, their friends and family will support their efforts to become free of drugs. But often—especially if your friends and acquaintances use drugs themselves—those around you might feel like you're rebuffing or judging them if you decide to make a change. As a result, some of these people might make your difficult change even harder to accomplish.

Once you decide to live a drug-free life, you may face many challenges that can interfere with your success. But *you're* the one who will ultimately decide whether you'll turn away from drugs. In this chapter, I'll discuss how to change your mind-set and your surroundings in order to improve your chances of success. In the next chapter, I'll talk about how you can turn to other people for help in putting almost addiction behind you.

Becoming drug free can fundamentally change your daily life, from how you deal with stress and anxiety, to the people you associate with, to how you spend your spare time. Deciding to make this change often brings on misgivings and bouts of second-guessing, and it's likely that you'll waver in your decision from time to time. This is both normal and expected, because people aren't likely to completely embrace changes that will drastically affect their lives without hesitation or second thoughts. Whether it's deciding whom to marry, which school to attend, which job to take (if you're lucky enough in this economy to have a choice!), or what car to buy, taking time to work through big changes is very, very common.

And learning to live your life without drugs can indeed take time. You probably won't be able to simply toss your remaining weed or pills or other drugs, vow to quit cold turkey, and never have a temptation to use or an actual relapse as long as you live.

Instead, you'll need to make relatively comprehensive changes to your entire life to support this decision. This requires working to improve your emotional, mental, and physical well-being in general. You must also understand the "triggers" in your life that prompt you to use drugs and think about how you might change them—or if you can't change them, how you might respond differently in the future instead of reaching for that next hit. You may also need to find other activities that spark your interest.

Developing new routines, confronting your triggers, perhaps finding new social circles, improving your health, and making other changes in your life does not guarantee that you'll remain free of drugs. But if you *don't* do these things, remaining drug free will be a much less realistic possibility, as Madeline's upcoming story illustrates.

Throughout the book, I have told patient stories that have illustrated the main points of each chapter. I wanted to do the same here, but—despite racking my brain to recall a case for this chapter—I simply couldn't think of a patient who'd successfully addressed almost addiction with no outside assistance. Then it finally occurred to me that I couldn't find an example because people who successfully tackle almost addiction on their own obviously don't avail themselves of my services, and thus never come to my attention. The people who see me realize they can't do it alone and have already reached out for help.

Because of this, the story I'm about to tell is different from those in the previous chapters. It offers a look at a woman who continued to smoke marijuana regularly despite my repeated encouragement to stop. In addition to trying to help her see how marijuana was harming her life, I also encouraged her—largely in vain—to make several changes in her life that might have helped her feel better about herself.

Although Madeline did not end up making these changes, hopefully you'll choose to do so.

Madeline's Story

When we first met, Madeline was in her mid-thirties, with a husband and three young children. She grew up in an affluent suburb of New York City with a mother who was cold and condescending. Her father adored her, but he worked long hours as a stock trader and left her mother to manage the day-to-day aspects of raising the kids.

Growing up, Madeline's self-esteem was always shaky—likely because of her mother's constant badgering—and she actively sought approval from friends and classmates. When she was a sophomore in high school, a couple of older boys encouraged her to drink alcohol, telling her that "all of the cool kids drink." She quickly became inebriated, at which point the boys began to remove her clothing and fondle her. She didn't remember everything that transpired after that, but the boys took Polaroid photos of her while she was naked and then began passing them around school. Within days, virtually the entire student body had seen the photos, which set off an avalanche of jokes, taunts, and overt humiliation. (No adults were ever told about what happened, and the boys were never punished for their behavior.)

Even though Madeline didn't engage in any consensual sexual activity until she was in college, her reputation as a "slut" stuck with her throughout high school. Almost twenty years later, her eyes still welled with tears any time she would recount this time of her life.

Madeline was delighted that in college she able to forge a new identity. She did well academically and had several long-term relationships with boys in college. Once she graduated, she worked a few years and then decided that she wanted to be a teacher, partly to help young people navigate the challenging years that had caused her so much pain. She went back to college to earn a master's degree in education. While there, she met her future husband, Joe, who was attending law school.

Joe didn't thrill Madeline, but he was a decent, kind man with a promising career ahead, so Madeline said yes to his proposal after they'd been dating for a year. They married just after he finished school and then moved so he could take a job in a midsize law firm. Madeline found a teaching job in a private high school, and they were off to a promising start as a couple.

Several months after they began their new jobs, Madeline unexpectedly became pregnant. But her husband, unsure that he'd even last at the firm for several years, much less ever make partner, didn't feel ready to have a child. He strongly pushed Madeline to have an abortion. Madeline reluctantly agreed to the procedure but immediately afterward felt like she'd made a horrible mistake.

Between the humiliation she endured as an adolescent and the guilt she felt for agreeing to the abortion, Madeline would often say that she didn't believe she deserved to have any happiness in her life because she was a horrible person.

Two years later, Madeline became pregnant again and this time carried the child to term and bore a son. Like many moms, she decided that raising her child was more meaningful to her than her job—even though she loved teaching—and she never returned to the school after her maternity leave. Within the next four years she gave birth to two more children. Meanwhile, Joe's work never relented, and although they were delighted when he eventually made partner in his law firm, he continued to work eighty to one hundred hours every week.

The outside world would see Madeline as a well-educated, devoted mother and a wife to an affluent white-collar professional. But as with every almost addicted person, her outside appearance is only part of her story.

Madeline first smoked marijuana in college. Throughout college and graduate school, she continued to smoke it but only occasionally. During her years as a teacher, she would smoke once or twice a month in the evenings while she was waiting for her husband to come home from work. Although he didn't use marijuana himself—he wasn't interested and was such a consummate lawyer that he strived hard to obey the law—he cared only a little that she did.

Her marijuana use escalated to one or two nights per week after she left the paid workforce. She would never smoke during the day or when she had any child care duties. She never got into any trouble as a result of her marijuana use.

Madeline consistently remarked that marijuana relaxed her, and it helped treat the shame she felt over the humiliating episode from her adolescence and the guilt she felt about the abortion. Madeline almost always smoked alone, and nobody outside of a few close friends and her husband knew that she used the drug.

Madeline had seen therapists off and on prior to coming to see me. In addition to chronic low self-esteem and depressed mood, Madeline suffered occasional panic attacks, often when she had to interact with her mother. Madeline felt like her kids "needed to know their grandparents," and because of this she maintained more contact with her mother than she would've preferred.

Madeline never saw her drug use as a problem, aside from the isolation it caused her to feel. Indeed, any time I raised it as an important issue, she would remind me of the very real emotional trauma she had suffered and tell me that marijuana helped her cope with all that she had endured. Even though she went to lengths to look "put together"—she dressed impeccably and frequently sported a new hairstyle—she was moderately overweight and rarely exercised. Her diet, as much as I could tell, was essentially standard meat and potatoes American fare. Although she was raised Presbyterian and considered herself a believer, other than baptizing her children, she hadn't attended church in more than a decade.

Any time I encouraged Madeline to take any step toward self-improvement—such as a little exercise, eating a better diet, attending church—she would either smile coyly or make excuses about why next month would be a better time to make a change.

In fact, Madeline might have done many things that could have improved her mood and mental well-being and probably (if not definitely) would have decreased her need to continue smoking marijuana. These steps could have helped her become more mentally and physically fit so that drug use would have held less appeal for her.

But she didn't take those steps. Let's take a look at them and see whether you might decide that these changes are worth making.

Discover Your Triggers—and Keep Away from Them

Even among people who are truly addicted to drugs and are trying to quit, overcoming physical dependence is just one aspect of kicking the drug. This physical dependence can produce extremely uncomfortable symptoms in some people when they try to stop using drugs.

Yet the physical dependence—that is, your body screaming out for just one more hit—is often not the hardest part of quitting, even for those with a true addiction. The more difficult aspect of quitting is often the habitual aspect of drug use.

What do I mean by this? Consider the tobacco smoker who has been smoking for twenty years. Unconsciously she lights up a cigarette as she opens the newspaper at breakfast, when she walks the dog, drives the car, takes a break at work, finishes dinner, and so on. She no longer even feels the cigarette dangling between her right index and middle fingers. But when it's not there, she notices its absence.

This is the aspect of cigarette use that is even tougher for many smokers to deal with than the physical addiction to nicotine. I had a patient several years ago who smoked two packs of cigarettes a day. I prescribed him a medication to help him kick the habit, and when we met three weeks later, he told me that the drug completely squelched his bodily cravings for tobacco and eliminated his physical desire to smoke. However, after several days of not smoking he realized he wasn't ready to give up smoking because the habit was too much a part of his everyday life.

Even *non*drug related activities are hard to quit once they become a habit. Imagine how you feel when you have to drive a different route to work than the one that's so familiar you can navigate it without your full attention. People who are deeply into running might feel agitated all day if they miss their morning jog. Couples who watch TV together every night might not easily come up with something else to do when the cable goes out. As they say, old habits die hard.

If you don't yet have a full-fledged addiction but are only almost addicted, you likely won't have much physical dependence on the drug. Instead, it's your daily routines that involve the drug that will probably push you more strongly to continue using. So once you realize it's time to stop using drugs, one of the first things you should do is come up with a list of all of the situations and events that may trigger you to crave a hit. These might include

- boredom
- loneliness
- fatigue
- physical pain
- painful memories
- routines with others, such as going to bars, concerts, or nightclubs
- an activity you do with your spouse or partner
- something you do after a fight with your spouse or partner
- a need to relax after work
- something you do when you're having trouble sleeping

Once you come up with a list of your triggers, write down what you'll do the next time each situation or feeling arises that doesn't involve taking a hit. If boredom or loneliness turns your thoughts to escaping through drugs, maybe you shouldn't come home to an empty apartment after work. Maybe you should stop at the gym or have a friend over for dinner instead.

If you inevitably discover that a night out clubbing just isn't the same without Ecstasy or other club drugs, perhaps it's time to find some other weekend activity. If you and your friend always smoke pot when she's in town, perhaps it's time to take a hiatus from this friendship. As you see, sometimes dealing with your triggers means you need to try something different. Here are a few suggestions.

Change Your Environment (Including the Drug-Using People in It)

Many of the patients I have worked with over the years who abuse drugs do so only in certain social situations and with a certain group of friends. Adolescents especially will often say "Everybody I know smokes weed." For some of them this may well be true . . . and if so it means they probably need to know different people.

I can't stress enough that for many, many people—especially if you mostly take drugs with friends—changing your habits means that you'll need to stop hanging out with certain people. Some true friends who use drugs will respect you if you're trying to remain clean, but many not-so-true "friends" who use drugs will feel like you're trying to make them look bad for their ongoing use. They'll encourage you to keep joining them so they feel better about what they're doing.

And even if these people are not directly encouraging you to use, it is very hard to be around a group of people you like and respect and not join them in an activity—*any* activity—in which they are all engaged. If all your friends love football and you don't, you're going to have trouble feeling like part of the group on Super Bowl day if you're reading a book while they're yelling at the TV. Although you might be able to refrain once or twice, expecting to stay drug free around friends who continue to use is not realistic.

Not surprisingly, then, research has confirmed that people's peers influence their behavior and their chances of developing a substance use disorder. One study found that associating with people who engage in "deviant behavior" increases the likelihood of later developing a substance use disorder. The researchers included lying, stealing, skipping school, destroying property, selling drugs, and attacking others in their list of deviant behaviors.[79] A large Finnish study also found that adolescents with peers who smoked tobacco or used drugs were more likely to use illicit drugs themselves.[80]

Since people are social creatures, it's only natural that the behavior of peers has an influence. It's natural to want to spend time with people who do things you enjoy. Because of this, if you're serious about getting off drugs, you should review your stable of friends. If they use drugs, you probably need to begin getting some distance from them.

But don't stop there. You don't want to cut what you found to be a fun, pleasurable section out of your life without filling in that space with something equally enjoyable. If you give up a drug and then your life becomes less interesting because you haven't replaced it with something better, you're going to be more likely to return to it. But if you replace the drug use with appealing people and activities, you're not going to have as much desire (or room in your life) to return to drugs later.

What could you do instead of using? Buy a musical instrument or dig out one you played earlier in life. Volunteer. Learn to cook or find another hobby. Travel, either in your area or abroad. Go online and find communities of people who get together to talk about or do something that appeals to you (Meetup.com is one website that helps people find others nearby who share similar interests).

When You're Drug-Free . . . But Your Partner Isn't

In my day-to-day work, I have seen countless instances of people deciding to get clean and sober—be it from alcohol or other drugs—and return home from detox or rehab to a spouse or partner who continues to use. Once home, some find living a drug-free life impossible to maintain. By contrast, I've seen married couples get clean and sober together and be tremendously supportive to one another in their attempts to remain drug free.

One 2010 study that followed 273 couples found that women whose husbands used prescription drugs had a higher risk of misusing these medications. Some evidence suggested that this risk was due to having the medications around, rather than the husband using them, per se.[81]

What can you do if you're trying to clean up your life and your partner isn't ready? That's a tough one—but it's wise to find a solution that gets your partner's drug use away from you. Options include

- ending the relationship
- asking your partner to limit any drug use to times and places when you're not around and to clear all drugs and drug paraphernalia out of the home
- finding an array of other activities to do with your partner if drug use has been an important part of your relationship
- helping your partner turn away from drugs so you can start living a drug-free life together

Anything you can do that isn't harmful to you or others and that either relieves stress or passes time in a drug-free manner is far preferable to using drugs.

Make a Plan

Changing almost any habit can be difficult. You might find it helpful to make a list of the reasons you want to quit (then if you ever wonder "Why am I doing this?" you have an easy way of reminding yourself). It might also help to make a list of the reasons why quitting won't necessarily be easy (so you can remind yourself, "Oh, right. I saw this complication coming"). Setting a specific date to quit or laying out a timeline to do so is probably also a good step to take. Start buying less of your drug—or better yet, simply don't buy any at all.

When you're serious about stopping, toss out your bongs, pipes, and other drug paraphernalia. Change your cell phone number. Delete your contact list. Don't pick up the phone when your dealer or a drug-using buddy is calling. Although this might seem selfish, so be it. When you need to make a change for the better, you should place your own needs ahead of what others want of you.

Once you begin to take action, be kind to yourself. Be prepared for setbacks. This is normal and expected, and you should try to focus on getting past the obstacles rather than getting down on yourself should you hit a few bumps along the way.

Move Your Body

Physical activity is excellent for overall health and well-being. It reduces fatigue, helps alleviate depression, and can get you out in public interacting with fit, healthy role models. Exercising regularly may also help you stay away from drugs. Some studies suggest that becoming more physically active can help decrease substance use and may serve as a useful addition to substance abuse treatment.[82]

A recently published pilot study from Denmark, for example, examined whether exercise affected drug behavior among individuals who were addicted to drugs. Thirty-eight people entered the study, which consisted of group exercise three times weekly for two to six months. Of the twenty subjects who completed the program, five had ceased all drug use, and ten reported that they were using less. Only four said their drug use had not changed. Overall, the participants reported having a better quality of life and more energy.[83]

Another 2010 study, this one from Spain, included 554 college students. The study found a connection between playing a sport and less substance use in the past month. Playing a sport also meant that individuals were less likely to be physically dependent on substances.[84]

Exercising early in life may also be linked to less drug use later. A study from Norway, for example, found that participation in team or endurance sports as an adolescent was related to less marijuana and tobacco use later in life, while a large Finnish twin study found that those who were inactive as adolescents were more likely to use drugs in adulthood.[85]

Just how does exercise affect substance use? The link is probably due to a number of factors. First, participating in sports takes time—time that might otherwise be spent finding and taking drugs. Also, those who play sports might be more interested in physical fitness in general and highly attuned to their bodies, and these traits may be protective against substance use.

As a result, readers who are almost addicted should consider taking up sports and other physical activities as they work to become drug-free. I've seen a number of patients who became more physically active as they were getting off drugs, sometimes with amazing results. Walking and jogging are ideal forms of exercise for someone who's been physically inactive. They're inexpensive and easy to do. Also, you can walk or jog with other people, and most communities offer races that range in length from 5K (5 kilometers or 3.1 miles) to marathons (26.2 miles). Some people find that they enjoy channeling the time and energy that would have gone to drugs into running such races instead.

However, although Madeline would occasionally vow to start going to a gym on a regular basis, for one reason or another she never managed to go more than twice before declaring defeat and retreating to her home and kids.

Clean Up Your Diet

One change that Madeline—and the rest of us—could benefit from would be to go Mediterranean. That doesn't mean hopping a plane to northern Italy, but rather eating a little more like people do in that part of the world.

By now the healthful effects of eating what is known as a Mediterranean diet are abundantly clear. Such a diet includes whole-grain bread and pasta, fresh vegetables, beans and legumes, and olive oil, which is high in monounsaturated fat (a kind of fat linked to heart health). Furthermore, this diet is light on red meat and moderately heavy on seafood.

Study after study has shown that eating these foods helps prevent heart disease, some forms of cancer, and diabetes. It can also bring about weight loss. Plus, new research on the Mediterranean diet is showing that it also can improve mood and overall well-being.

For example, a 2009 study from Spain, in which participants were followed for about four years, concluded that this diet may be protective against depression.[86] In another study from 2011 using the same group of participants, researchers found that following a Mediterranean diet was associated with improved overall mental health, including feelings of vitality and improved social functioning.[87]

Another randomized, controlled trial from Australia published in 2011 drew a similar conclusion about the healthful effects of eating a Mediterranean diet. Participants who were asked to follow the Mediterranean diet reported significant improvements in vigor, alertness, and contentment compared to those who didn't change their eating habits. Unlike the two Spanish studies, this study found these positive effects *after only ten days* of the diet.[88]

To my knowledge, no research directly links the Mediterranean diet to a lower tendency toward using or abusing drugs, so it would be a huge stretch to draw any direct conclusions. But given the amount of research that has found a connection between feeling better about oneself and decreased substance use, I feel safe in stating that eating a healthier diet can lead to an overall improvement in one's mental state, which in turn might contribute to decreased substance abuse.

In Madeline's case, I was never able to convince her to alter her eating in any significant way, so we didn't get to find out whether she would have felt better had she decided to eat differently.

Address Your Other Bad Habits Too

Bad habits often run together. When people use drugs, they are more likely to also smoke and drink. Want proof? Consider one Canadian study from 2006 involving 149 drug-using college students, which found that alcohol, tobacco, and marijuana were frequently used together.[89] The large Spanish study of 554 college students, cited earlier, also found that using tobacco significantly increased the chances that someone would use marijuana, pills, and other illegal drugs. According to the study, consuming alcohol increased the odds that someone was also abusing tobacco and marijuana.

Although I could cite many more studies, my main point is that if you are serious about quitting drugs, giving up some of your other bad habits at the same time may improve your chance of success. Fortunately, many of the steps toward conquering your almost addiction to illicit drugs (like exercising more and avoiding situations where you use) may also help you turn away from alcohol and tobacco.

Tend to Your Spiritual Life

If a patient has religious beliefs and is trying to get free of drugs, I will often strongly encourage him to become more spiritually active.

Spirituality and religious belief can enhance some measurements of overall physical well-being.[90] But even beyond a general sense of well-being, religious activity is associated with better outcomes among those who've had problems with drugs. One 2007 study that included 169 people who sought treatment for opiate or cocaine abuse found that participants who said they frequently spent time on religious and/or spiritual activities were more likely to remain in treatment and use fewer drugs.[91]

In the next chapter, I'll discuss how your pastor or other clergyperson—if you care to open up to such a person and ask for assistance—can be a valuable ally in your recovery from almost addiction.

Even if you aren't religious, developing a sense of a higher purpose—a power greater than yourself that gives meaning to your life—can fill the void that you may be currently trying to fill with drugs. That may be your family and friends, community, a cause that addresses some social or other need in the world, or all of the above.

Look for a Job or Other Meaningful Activity

For many people with drug-related issues, work is protective in various ways. Work is usually a *social* experience—it surrounds you with other people. In most cases, going to work means you have to groom yourself adequately, show up someplace on a regular basis, and answer to others (even if that means just obeying general norms of social conduct and at times needing to explain your motives and actions). Even though some aspects of work can be a chore, most of them are conducive to mental health and well-being.

In my daily life and psychiatric practice, I've seen more than a few people who were wealthy enough that they didn't have to work. And among these individuals, I've seen more than a little mental health disruption. In one instance, an Ivy League–educated man told me that he "needed to get a job" because he was going out of his mind with nothing to do all day. I've also seen equally intelligent folks turn to drinking and drugs to pass the time, becoming ever more eccentric because their money allowed them to not have to interact with the public like everyone else.

Research has consistently shown that having a job is associated with better outcomes for people who abuse drugs. So if you're trying to kick drugs and you don't presently have a job, think about checking out the "Help Wanted" ads. Finding employment isn't as easy as snapping your fingers, of course, so if it takes a bit longer than you'd like, consider volunteering somewhere until a regular job opens up. In Madeline's case, she could have gotten back into teaching and volunteered in a classroom or an after-school program while she waited to get a classroom of her own.

If Possible, Wait to Have Sex for the First Time

Okay, odds are good that this advice is coming to you too late. Nonetheless, I'm including this tidbit not because I think I'm going to influence anyone to actually delay becoming sexually active, but more as a teaching point.

Research is fairly clear and consistent in concluding that people who have intercourse for the first time later in life are less likely to abuse drugs.[92] Now, I don't think that this relationship is *causal*—that is, I don't think there is something intrinsic to having sex later in life that leads one to also abstain from drugs. Instead, these factors go hand in hand, and it's not hard to imagine why.

Most individuals who choose to hold off on sexual activity until later in life are more cautious and careful and more prone to follow the rules, and those same qualities also lead people to be less likely to use or abuse drugs.

Now might be a good time to look at other risky behaviors in your life: speeding, not wearing a seatbelt, having sexual relationships that are ill advised, and off-the-cuff investment decisions, for example. Perhaps you'd be better off taking fewer of these risks or channeling them into less hazardous activities.

How to Make the Best Use of Your Own Resources

- Examine what triggers your drug use (like loneliness, boredom, certain situations), and learn how to avoid those triggers or cope with them in other ways.

- Set a date to quit—and stick to it.

- Eat a diet that's heavy in fresh fruits and vegetables, whole grains, and lean meat, with a minimum of junk food and fast food.

- Exercise at least thirty minutes most days, and consider seeking out team sports (like a volleyball or softball league through your workplace).

- Look for a job if you're not currently employed.

- Consider dropping friends who abuse drugs, or at a minimum spend less time with them.

- Avoid bars or parties where drugs are likely to be present.

- If you're inclined toward religious belief and practice, get into the habit of going to services regularly.

Madeline's Outcome

Madeline never stopped using marijuana during the three years we worked together. She continued to smoke it mostly because she didn't see any major downsides to doing so, and the drug calmed and soothed her and occupied her time.

She'd long ago given up on trying to get fit. Reentering the workforce never really crossed her mind, in part because she figured she'd fail whatever drug test she might have to take, since marijuana can stay in your system for weeks. And although she followed the news closely, she had few hobbies or outside interests. Instead of surrounding herself with people who didn't use drugs, she isolated herself in a party of one, surrounded by smoke.

Madeline didn't take any action to improve her odds of ever escaping marijuana, so it's not surprising that she continued to smoke regularly.

■ ◆ ■

9

Time for a Change
Getting Help from Others

By and large, human nature resists change.

Perhaps you can look to physics again for a clue as to why this is so: Isaac Newton's first law of motion states (and I'm paraphrasing) that an object at rest will tend to stay at rest unless it's acted upon by an external force. Simply put, inertia is the norm. If you apply this law to human behavior, that means it's hard to bring about change in oneself unless there is a compelling reason to do so.

You can see this in all areas of life. Think of all the overweight people who find it seemingly impossible to lose any weight and then keep it off. Or the woman who needs to leave a psychologically abusive boyfriend, but just can't seem to find her way to the door once and for all. Or the person who's chronically late. Or the person who can't stop nail biting. Or smoking. Or eating junk food.

The same is true for people who are almost addicted to a drug. A bystander might assume that quitting would be straightforward, especially when you are not truly addicted and won't experience physical withdrawal symptoms. But the reality is that bringing about change—any change, for anyone—can be daunting. Frequently, people make several failed attempts at quitting before they succeed.

In the end, one person is at the center of an almost addiction—you, the person who is almost addicted—and quitting is ultimately up to you. That said, you are not alone in your struggle to turn away from drugs; in fact, you are likely to have many avenues of support and assistance, including your loved ones, medical and mental health professionals, and members of the clergy.

Some folks will be able to get clean on their own without any major outside support, although these individuals are rare. Others might need only to reach out to one outside source for support. Still others, like my patient Kaylo, look to a number of different resources for help. As with the other real-life stories you've read throughout this book, Kaylo's experience highlights the perils of almost addiction. But it also provides an example of the many people who turn away from almost addiction every day.

Kaylo's Story

I first met Kaylo nearly a decade ago when he was in his mid-thirties. He was a college-educated Nigerian who had immigrated to the United States roughly six years before I met him. Kaylo was also a devout Christian. When he first came to America, he began working in a convenience store as a clerk. It didn't take long for the store owner to realize how bright Kaylo was and to promote him to manager.

Kaylo was married, but his wife—who was also Nigerian—had overstayed her visa and in the years following the September 11 terror attack on the World Trade Center was deported. Kaylo told me that she was living in England and was perpetually trying to get back to the States, although her prospects seemed nil. Kaylo was uncertain if or when he'd see his wife again.

Until shortly before our meeting, Kaylo had never seen a psychiatrist or therapist for any reason, nor had he ever thought about suicide prior to that time. He said he also had never drunk more than a tiny amount of alcohol or used any drugs whatsoever. But things changed dramatically for Kaylo several months before I met him.

Losing his job after an accounting oversight may have been the event that set his psychiatric saga in motion. Although he was never happy about his wife being kept out of the United States, with more time on his hands following his job loss, he started feeling despondent that he might not see her again. That's when Kaylo started smoking crack cocaine.

And with that, he came to feel like his "life was over" and that he had no reason for living. He repeatedly told me that his family became angry with him for his drug use, as well as his problems that they considered largely of his own making. He began scouting out buildings from which he could jump. Because of his depression and suicidal feelings, Kaylo was hospitalized several times in the months before I met him. He couldn't commit to staying alive and kept telling people he wanted to die.

At our first few meetings, Kaylo sometimes reported having auditory hallucinations—hearing things that weren't really there. If he was feeling especially bad, he'd admit to using crack once or twice since our previous meeting. If life felt somewhat better, he would tell me that he managed to remain drug free. Sometimes, no doubt, he told me he wasn't using any cocaine, when in fact he was. (Whereas many psychiatrists get unhappy when their patients lie to them, for the most part I expect it. After all, how many people find it easy to tell their innermost secrets to someone who is virtually a complete stranger?)

Several times during the first year and a half that we worked together, Kaylo needed to be admitted to a psychiatric ward because he was planning to kill himself. During one of these inpatient stays, he tried to asphyxiate himself by placing a plastic bag over his head. The nurses happened to walk into his room and saved him.

Not long after this hospital stay, Kaylo missed an appointment with me. (In the clinic where I see Kaylo, it is not uncommon for patients to miss appointments, and I usually don't immediately try to track down patients to find out why.) When I realized over the next several weeks that Kaylo was still out of touch, I tried calling his cell phone. The call went straight to voice mail, which said his mailbox was full and not accepting any more messages. I found his brother's name in his chart as an emergency contact, so I called him. When I asked for Kaylo, I got this curt reply: "Kaylo's dead," followed by an abrupt click.

I felt terrible, waited a few minutes to take in what I'd just heard, and decided to call back to try to get more information. I called the number again several more times, but my calls went to voice mail. I remembered hearing several days earlier that someone had jumped off a hotel that spans the Massachusetts Turnpike just outside of Boston, and I suspected it was Kaylo.

I broke the news to the team when we met several days later. People were saddened to hear of Kaylo's death, but not shocked, given the persistence of his cocaine use and depression.

Then, imagine my surprise three weeks later when I walked into the waiting area of my clinic and there sat Kaylo—very much alive—who hoped he could talk to me even though he didn't have an appointment. I was busy, but made time to meet with him. He told me that several weeks earlier he left a suicide note for his family, drove off to an isolated spot, and overdosed on Tylenol.

A bystander saw him and called for help, and the paramedics brought him to an emergency room. There, his stomach was pumped and Kaylo was admitted yet again to a psychiatric unit. Since he didn't have his cell phone or any form of identification on him and initially he wouldn't give health care workers his name, his family didn't know about his admission and assumed the worst.

This suicide attempt ultimately proved to be a turning point for Kaylo. Although he remained depressed and continued to use cocaine in moments of weakness and despair, he gradually began to improve on multiple fronts. He eventually decided he wasn't ever going to live with his wife again, and he filed for divorce. He managed to land a new job. He also resumed regular church attendance and began to discuss his problems with his minister. Although his family was quite upset with him for his drug use, he eventually began to make amends with them and they allowed him back into the fold.

Kaylo moved past his almost addiction and, in a way, came back from the dead.

Getting Help from Your Doctor

In chapter 5, I noted some of the reasons that primary care doctors may miss cases of almost addiction. Let's make clear that they're more likely to overlook cases *if it's up to them to discover them.* When doctors have only ten to twenty minutes to delve into a single problem you bring them, let alone give you a general checkup, almost addiction isn't likely to catch their attention if you don't mention it or show an obvious sign of drug use.

But if you do mention the problem and ask for help, any competent primary care doctor is going to listen to your description and address your concerns.

Because your primary care doctor knows your medical history, this is often a good place to start when seeking help for an almost addiction. One issue your doctor will be concerned about—which might surprise you—is whether the drug use has caused any damage to your body. If you smoke pot habitually, how is your lung function? If you use cocaine, how does your heart sound?

Most people find little to no embarrassment in visiting a primary care physician, whereas you might feel that seeing a substance abuse counselor, a psychiatrist, or a mental health worker in general carries a huge stigma. As such, a primary care office is often the first stop for people who believe they might have a problem with their substance use.

If you don't have a primary care doctor—and many people don't—now is a good time to find one. The doctor could be a family practice physician, an internist, or for women an OB/GYN or for seniors a geriatrician. If you're a teenager, you might be comfortable with a doctor who specializes in adolescent medicine. These doctors spend a large chunk of their day discussing drug and alcohol use, sex, and other issues that relate to teen health.

As part of their general medical training, most primary care physicians learn how to use certain screening tools, or questionnaires, to assess substance use. In a primary care setting, screening for addiction might include initially asking whether the patient has consumed alcohol or other intoxicating substances during the last year. If the answer is no, the screen is complete. If the answer is yes, then the primary care physician should use additional screening tools to sort out a possible substance abuse problem. Designed to be easy to implement and quick to use, these tools will often help sort out the extent of the substance abuse problem—that is, whether the person is likely addicted or is somewhere in the almost addicted realm. An example of one of these screening tools is the DAST that you saw in the first chapter.

This is important: if the screening tools verify that you don't meet all the criteria for addiction, don't let the doctor—or yourself—pronounce you in the free and clear. Even drug use that wouldn't be considered an addiction is still a problem, and it's a reason for you to ask your doctor to start offering solutions.

A so-called brief intervention and advice from the doctor may be all the solution that you need to help you lick your problem. A brief intervention may just consist of several key items of information, along with a strong suggestion that you decrease your use. Is this type of very simple intervention really effective? The short answer is yes.

Brief interventions have been studied mostly in relation to alcohol use, and to a lesser extent for drugs other than alcohol, and indeed they can result in improved outcomes. One study found that simply providing regular amphetamine users with a self-help booklet along with two to four counseling sessions resulted in better outcomes for abstinence from amphetamines.[93] Another found that a brief intervention consisting of a single interaction in the clinic reduced cocaine and heroin use even after six months.[94] Furthermore, a Canadian study concluded that participating in nothing more than an assessment and brief intervention led to a reduction in illicit drug use, which in turn resulted in fewer adverse consequences from the substance use, as well as more confidence in the ability to avoid drugs several months later.[95]

The upshot is that even if a medical professional does little more than offer brief counseling, you will be more likely to kick your almost addiction and move forward with your life. It's not that the intervention magically does all the work. You showing a willingness to seek help may serve as a sign that you're ready to take the other actions necessary for stopping your drug use, like confronting the underlying problems that you've been trying to address with drugs or staying away from situations and friends who make your drug use more likely.

But it's also possible that a visit or two to a primary care doctor will not suffice. Your doctor may want to refer you to a mental health worker, a psychiatrist who specializes in addiction, or an addiction counselor. Or perhaps your doctor has a colleague in internal or family practice medicine who subspecializes in addiction, and she will refer you there. In addition, she might encourage you to begin attending Alcoholics Anonymous (AA) or Narcotics Anonymous (NA) meetings. If a drug problem is worrisome enough—and this usually would not be the case with the almost addicted—a referral to a treatment facility might be indicated. This course of action might be warranted in someone who uses drugs infrequently but does so in high-risk situations such as caring for patients or teaching young children.

In Kaylo's case, his primary care physician certainly knew of his travails with crack cocaine and monitored him medically to be alert for physical damage from the drug. Kaylo was young, and although cocaine is never entirely safe given how it affects the body, he never suffered too much physically as a result of his use of crack.

Getting Help from a Mental Health Provider

Any psychiatrist, psychologist, or therapist should be knowledgeable about substance use disorders of any kind, since the overlap between substance abuse and mental health issues is so high. For example, one report several years ago stated that as many as 40 to 60 percent of people who come to mental health settings also have a substance use diagnosis, and that 60 to 80 percent of individuals entering substance abuse facilities have a co-occurring mental illness diagnosis.[96] If one were to include those who are almost addicted, that number would no doubt be substantially higher. As a result, most professionals in the mental health field constantly work with individuals who have substance use disorders, and they should be valuable resources for you.

Your mental health practitioner should be nonjudgmental and should try to learn as much as possible about your relationship to substances. This provider's overall approach should be to ask questions about your substance use, provide feedback about the risks of that use, emphasize personal responsibility for changing the behavior, and offer advice about cutting down or stopping drug use. My advice for you is to keep your appointments and be as honest as you can when answering questions or talking about your problematic relationship to drugs.

This general framework provides what is known as motivational interviewing, which is one form of a brief intervention. The professional will likely try to follow the DARES approach. This begins with an attempt to do the following:[97]

- **Develop** a discrepancy between what you say you want for yourself and how your current drug use could get in the way of achieving those goals.

- **Avoid** argumentation.

- **Roll** with resistance, because so much of drug use—even by those in the almost addicted realm—is characterized by denial ("It's not really causing any problems. I'm not really using that much."). The clinician should therefore be nonconfrontational and not push back if you display resistance, because it serves little purpose for a clinician to try to insist that the patient see how bad the drug use is for him.

- **Express** empathy.

- **Support** self-efficacy. This means you feel like the mental health professional is on your side, working with you as a teammate to steer you in the right direction, but is also giving you the tools you need to get out from under the burden of almost addiction using your own resources and determination. In motivational interviewing, the clinician and the person using substances set a course together for change. The client knows that she is in control and can make decisions for herself.

If your provider takes this approach, as he or she should, you will feel empowered to take control of your own course. You shouldn't feel guilty about any hesitations or qualms that arise while trying to change your behavior. Resistance to change is *normal* and should be expected. Don't feel bad if you feel this way—and don't tolerate a professional who can't accept that you may not move smoothly and swiftly away from drug use!

If you have any doubts about the value of seeing a professional to improve your chances of becoming drug free, know that the research clearly shows a link between seeking professional help and decreased use of drugs among those who've had drug-use issues.

Mental health treatment goes further than merely reducing drug use. It can also reduce some of the problems related to the drug use. One recent study found that among offenders who were participating in court-mandated drug treatment, the number of rearrests was lower among those who had received more treatment services and longer treatment length.[98]

The reason that professional help reduces drug use is no doubt multifactorial. But at a minimum, the individual who does reach out for professional help is probably more motivated

When to Go It Alone and When to Seek a Pro

While the list below is not hard and fast, it provides a general framework for deciding whether to confront your almost addiction alone or to seek professional help.

Reasons to Not Seek Professional Assistance Right Away

- You're suspicious of the fields of medicine or psychiatry.

- You are deeply religious and more apt to listen to your family or a clergyperson than to any mental health professional.

- You resent having a person of authority tell you what you should do.

- Despite reading everything in this book, you are still convinced that your drug use has caused no problems in your life. (If this is true, I would hope that you change your mind sooner rather than later, since almost addiction can definitely lead to life-changing consequences for you tomorrow, next year, or years from now.)

Reasons to Run to a Pro as Soon as Possible

- Something vital to your well-being—like your job or marriage—is in jeopardy because of your drug use, or you've already had a major consequence (like a car wreck) and you still can't stop using.

- You feel yourself becoming physically dependent on a substance (for example, you feel uneasy or sick when it's not in your system).

- You are beginning to feel like you can't live without a substance.

- You've gone the self-help route already but you're still using.

- Your drug use is harming your physical health.
- Your personal support network or family is unhappy with you or otherwise incapable of helping (or most of the people around you are using drugs too).
- You believe that you're more likely to listen to a trained professional than a layperson.

to stop using than somebody who doesn't. And that, combined with the expertise the professional brings to the table, greatly improves the odds of staying clean.

Kaylo made extensive use of psychiatric services, partly because he had such significant mental distress in addition to his cocaine use. But Kaylo's drug use compounded his distress by causing him to blow through whatever money he'd saved, which further alienated him from his family, who despised drugs. The treatment he received was therefore "dual diagnosis" in nature, which means it is appropriate for and addresses both substance use and psychiatric problems.

If you also have depression, anxiety, or other mental health concerns or life difficulties, your provider can help you deal with these as well. In addition to offering talk therapy for certain conditions or situations, a psychiatrist or other mental health care provider can help ensure that you receive necessary medication, which hopefully will be nonaddictive or non-habit forming.

One of my patients who was distraught about the lack of intimacy in her long-term relationship drank alcohol excessively in an attempt to avoid confronting her relationship problems head-on. I urged her for several years to go into couples counseling, so she could learn to directly deal with the issues at hand. Sure enough, when she finally entered couples therapy, her alcohol use fell sharply.

Taking Twelve Steps to Freedom from Drugs

Although you might think you have to be addicted or an alcoholic to attend AA or NA meetings (in part because in many of these meetings individuals introduce themselves by saying, "My name is _____ and I am an alcoholic"), that's not the case. Furthermore, some people also think that if they continue to use drugs, they are not welcome to attend these support group meetings. That's not true either. The only requirement for membership in AA or NA is that you must have a *desire* to stop using substances. There are closed meetings for people who self-identify as alcoholics and addicts, but anyone can go to open meetings without having to say you're an alcoholic or addict.

Whether you're *addicted* to drugs or *almost* addicted to drugs, you can gain an infinite amount of wisdom from attending these meetings. Research has shown that, all other things being equal, AA attendance is associated with better results for abstinence from intoxicating substances.

AA and its sister organization NA outline a path of self-illumination in which individuals not only acknowledge their lack of power over the drug they use, but also take stock of everything they've done that they regret or that has caused pain to those around them. This process is called taking a "fearless moral inventory." Once an individual starts, he's expected to make amends to those he has harmed, provided that making amends won't cause further pain and suffering to the individual receiving the apology (for example, it would be better not to apologize to the spouse of someone you had an affair with if the spouse isn't aware of the affair).

This process forces you to examine your life, including the things that have happened to you as a child or adult and the choices you've made. Since drug use doesn't occur in a vacuum —many factors play a role in your almost addiction, including these outside events and your own behaviors and thought processes—understanding all of these pieces is important for controlling or stopping your drug use.

AA is also a spiritually based approach, because it emphasizes the need to submit yourself to a Higher Power. You don't have to be a churchgoing person or even be religious to buy into this notion; you just have to accept that your own interests aren't at the center of the universe and that everyone has to answer to someone or something other than themselves.

Having a Higher Power is important for individuals who have had trouble with drugs because the pull of the drug can be so great that it takes over as a force in their lives. When it's time to move forward on another path, finding some other power is crucial. And rejecting the notion that you are in control of the drug is essential to overcoming its pull.

Accepting the Higher Power notion in Alcoholics Anonymous and Narcotics Anonymous is certainly a sticking point for some who contemplate giving up drugs in the program, but this need not keep you from attending such meetings. There are many groups in which Higher Power is not assumed to be synonymous with God but instead takes on a nonreligious aspect. Many members view their Higher Power as the Twelve

Step program itself. Any medium-size community or larger will offer many types of meetings—smoking or nonsmoking, same gender or not, and so on—including whether they are more religiously focused or not.

For those who simply can't stomach the idea of a Higher Power, even one that does not refer to God, it may be best to check out an alternative support network called Smart Recovery; much smaller than AA and NA, it offers group meetings that emphasize science and rationality and does not employ any concept of a Higher Power. There aren't as many meetings available so check to see if there's a Smart Recovery or other non–Twelve Step peer support group in your area.

One of the most powerful elements of AA is that it is a fellowship of individuals, and as such the group provides significant support to its members. This aspect of AA is vital to its success. Being in a group of others who readily admit their weakness and fallibility gives people permission to drop their own pretense of always being in control and of always making the right decisions. This sharing takes place in an atmosphere of trust—"What is said here, stays here"—and where "cross-talk" (interrupting or giving unsolicited advice) is discouraged. Sharing occurs in a circle of people who are in the same situation and who have made a commitment to listen to and support each other. For people who are addicted to alcohol or other drugs, having a sponsor—a person with some years of sobriety and experience who is willing to offer guidance and help in working the Twelve Step program—provides additional support.

Furthermore, much of AA involves individuals sharing their stories with one another—stories of the pain and suffering caused by their relationship to alcohol or other drugs. Stories like these convey morals and advice without seeming preachy or forceful. Research has shown that the community of supportive individuals found in AA can actually be more effective at helping people who are addicted or almost addicted remain substance free than support from other people in their life. "The type of social support specifically given by AA members, such as 24-hour availability, role modeling and experientially based advice for staying sober, may help to explain AA's mechanism of action," the researchers wrote.[99]

I'm not surprised at this finding, because often one's family has experienced so much pain by the actions of the person using drugs that, even though they deeply want the individual to get help and get clean, they may be too emotionally wounded to wholeheartedly offer support and guidance toward recovery. As a result, support from strangers who are personally unaffected by the individual's drug use can be more straight forward, as it comes without the baggage of being personally burned by the person who is almost addicted.

A question that may be a big concern for you right now is, How often would I need to go? The answer depends on your various personal needs and qualities. For someone who is truly addicted and coming out of an inpatient treatment program, the usual expectation is that the person will do "ninety in ninety," meaning ninety meetings in ninety days. That person will then find a "home group" to attend regularly, as well as going to other meetings periodically—most people attend anywhere from two to three meetings a week. For someone who is almost addicted, the need to attend meetings is probably less, although I certainly might recommend one to two meetings per week initially, but that is up to you and your situation.

Is this a lifelong commitment for someone who is almost addicted? Probably not. Many people with true addiction, no matter how long they've been clean, forever see themselves as addicts and so they do attend meetings indefinitely. On the other hand, I've known plenty who will tell me of an overpowering addiction to some substance a decade or two ago, but who don't identify as addicted anymore (though they in all likelihood would still be vulnerable to their former substance of abuse should they try it again).

If you're almost addicted, I would not speculate whether or not you'll need AA over the long term, but instead simply go to some meetings to see what you gain from the experience. Keep in mind that individual meetings can vary widely in their nature and composition, so if you go to a meeting and don't care for it, do not assume that all meetings are just like it; try another one. It's important to find a group that you're comfortable in— that is, one that has the right mix of people and the right structure for you (some meetings have speakers, whereas others go around the room and have members share on a topic, discuss how their week has gone, or talk about one of the Steps).

Should people who are almost addicted forever identify themselves as such? That depends on the individual, and it probably also depends on the extent to which she felt vulnerable to and harmed by the drug.

Getting Help from a Clergy Member

Many people define themselves by their religious faith, and the faithful can and do include abstainers, people who are almost addicted, people who abuse drugs, and those who are addicted. If your faith is important to you, then be sure not to overlook the support and guidance available from someone in the clergy or someone else from your religious community.

Apart from consulting a pastor or priest, consider pastoral counseling. A pastoral counselor provides psychologically sound therapy that weaves in the religious and spiritual dimension. This type of counseling can be remarkably effective because the client and the pastor can assume that one another shares a basic set of beliefs and values to a higher degree than in other professional relationships. Of course, merely sharing the same religion doesn't ensure that your beliefs will completely overlap, but the trust that is present initially can be lifesaving for some.

When pastoral counseling is done well, it can motivate the client to change in a nurturing and supportive way. Indeed, research has found that people who use drugs who frequently spend time on religious or spiritual activities have significantly better outcomes on reducing their drug use than those who do not.[100]

Good pastoral counselors or clergy will understand that it is up to the individual to get better and stay away from drugs, but they will also likely invoke God or a Higher Power as a source of assistance in getting clean and sober.

The best advice from such an individual will be that God will support you in becoming and staying drug free. However, reasonable pastoral counselors will invoke God and religion as a support, but not more. They will not claim that God will reward your good behavior and punish you for bad behavior. Why? Because although many "good" people do well and succeed in this life, many evil people also get ahead in the world.

Thus, even though it might seem natural for a member of the clergy to suggest that God will reward good behavior, the fact is that fate is random. Plenty of devout believers suffer pains of various kinds.

In Kaylo's case, although he initially had trouble being honest with those around him, he eventually told everyone what he was struggling with and became very forthcoming about his drug use, especially to his minister. In turn, his minister refrained from judging him and instead nurtured and supported Kaylo's efforts in remaining abstinent from drugs. In this way, his minister appropriately treated Kaylo's drug use as a problem to be solved, not as a moral failing or sinful behavior. In my experience, this attitude is optimal for addressing substance use of any sort.

Turning to Friends or Mentors

Opening up to someone you're close to and suggesting that you could use help and support might sound like a simple thing to do, but it often is surprisingly difficult. (It is hard enough for most people to admit to themselves that their drug use might be a problem.)

My caution to anyone who is considering opening up to a friend is to be sure that you will not be judged by this person. I can't emphasize this point enough. Even if you feel like you've done bad things, or maybe that you're a "bad" person, you don't need punishment right now. Don't compound your problem by reaching out to someone who is going to make matters worse by judging you.

You might have a problem, but it is not a *moral* problem. Nor is it a personal failing for which you should have shame or guilt piled on you. If you are going to reach out to a friend or mentor, that individual should have enough maturity to not subject you to a bunch of mindless platitudes: "God only gives you as much of a burden as you can handle," "Everything happens for a reason," and so on. The person should also be willing and ready to pitch in to help you kick your almost addiction.

One benefit of choosing this path is that you already know the person cares and will be supportive. A potential problem, ironically, is that a person who is close to you might feel desperate to do something to help but also be too close to make good, objective decisions. Also, if you care about your friend so much that you feel compelled to turn away from drugs in order to help alleviate his distress, then you might want to seek help elsewhere. Being in any kind of mental distress is hard enough, whether it's due to substance use or other emotional challenges, and feeling a need to appear happier or healthier than you are puts an additional burden on you.

Getting Help from Others: A Review

People all around you—in your family, social circles, church, and community—can help steer you away from drugs and keep you on a path that's far away from your almost addiction. Different people can offer different tools, but no one source of help may be able to offer you all that you need to get and stay drug free. Here's a quick recap of how to make the best use of outside help:

- **If you choose to see a mental health provider**, take the time to find someone knowledgeable about substance abuse issues who shares your values and communicates well with you and whose advice you think you'll respect.

- **If you reach out to your family**, especially if your family has been burned in some way by your drug use, hope for support and assistance, but don't be surprised if they are skeptical of your ability to change and quick to blame you for ongoing drug issues or related problems. If they are having trouble immediately giving you the help you need, try to not let this hamper your progress.

- **Seek out friends and acquaintances** who will not judge you for your substance use, but who instead will take on the attitude of rolling up their sleeves and helping you move forward until you're out of trouble. These need to be people you can call on even at inconvenient times. They should be there to help fill a need that you'd otherwise been trying to fill with a drug (or friends who use drugs or situations where drugs would be available). They need to provide an alternative to drug use.

- **Seeking help from clergy or a pastoral counselor** can be a terrific option for people who are moderately or strongly religious. That said, be wary of anyone who portrays your problem as a moral failing or sin. Almost addiction is a problem to be addressed and dealt with as quickly as possible, period!

- **AA or NA attendance** is associated with better outcomes for people who abuse substances, and it will also likely result in a better chance of success for people who are almost addicted. Because many in AA or NA have "been there themselves," they can give you excellent guidance and support.

- **Beware of platitudes**, which are clichéd bits of "wisdom" that do you no good. You shouldn't hear them from health care professionals or in the halls of AA or NA (though you occasionally might). However, you should expect them from those close to you if they are not mental health professionals or otherwise well versed in substance use disorders. If someone is just giving you worn-out advice of the sort that you'd see embroidered on a wall hanging, you may want to turn elsewhere for a listening ear.

Kaylo's Outcome

With the exception of a few slips that didn't lead him seriously astray, Kaylo has stayed drug free for the past four years. He slowly ventured back into the work world and is now steadily employed. As he became healthier, he relied on many different sources of support, primarily his siblings, his minister, me, and his new wife. He says that he has remained completely forthcoming with all of these people and tells them everything that's going on in his life. His faith is stronger than ever.

Interestingly, Kaylo never felt the need to attend AA or NA meetings. I encouraged him to do so several times but never pushed the issue, mostly because he had such a strong personal and religious network and was so committed to coming in for psychiatric care.

Because his life has settled down dramatically, at our meetings we've had occasion to talk about world events as well as US politics—as opposed to managing one psychiatric crisis after another—and I am consistently struck by Kaylo's linguistic abilities, breadth of knowledge, and experience. When I asked him if he'd mind my relaying his story in this book, he replied, "No problem. You can even use my real name." Despite that offer, both his name and many of the identifying details of his story are changed, as such details are in all of the stories in this book.

Kaylo's new wife recently gave birth to a daughter, whom he adores. He says he feels great and has no desire to use drugs again.

❖

10

After Almost Addiction—Now What?
Living without Drugs

Let's suppose that you have taken everything to heart that you have read in this book so far. Using the tools and advice in the previous chapters, you not only stop using drugs, but also commit to remaining drug free. You pass up the next hit that comes along, then go a day, then a week, then a month without using.

What happens then? Staying away from drugs—assuming you're not in prison or otherwise simply unable to procure them—is often only possible when you create a new and different approach to your life. Being drug free is important, but it is unlikely to happen if you're not otherwise living a fulfilling and healthy life.[101]

When people talk about being in "recovery" from substance dependence, they're referring to both remaining drug free and to being engaged in a productive life with a focus on overall health and well-being. They realize that drug use didn't just occur on its own—it developed as a result of other negative elements in their lives. Now they have the wisdom to not only root out the weeds of drug use, but to relandscape their lives so new weeds can't spring up again.

People who have had substance abuse problems and are incarcerated or unable to obtain their drug of abuse haven't necessarily changed. In medicine or in the halls of AA, these folks may be called "dry drunks," because they retain all of the habits and troubling behaviors they had while they were using drugs, even if they haven't touched them in years.

Once you turn away from drugs, you can take a number of additional actions to stay on the path to recovery and a more fulfilling and rewarding life. That's what Ernesto did.

Ernesto's Story

Ernesto was a fast-rising architect in his first year out of architecture school. Newly married, he was working at one of the most prestigious architecture firms in the northeast.

And when we first met, he was not at all happy to be in my office.

Throughout most of the interview, he kept a flat, cold demeanor and answered my questions curtly and with few words. It was as though he were talking to me with his middle finger raised the whole time.

Several days earlier, his wife and one of his siblings confronted Ernesto and told him they were concerned that he was snapping and yelling much more than usual—and had simply become plain mean. They had figured out that he was using cocaine—although they didn't know how much—and insisted he get help.

Ernesto's wife had originally called my office on his behalf, telling me that she "barely recognized the man she knew a year earlier." She's the one who scheduled the first meeting. At that meeting, Ernesto admitted to using cocaine but said he only did it rarely and never at work or around his family. Regarding other substance use, Ernesto told me that he never had a problem with alcohol. In addition, he said he'd smoked marijuana a handful of times but that it had never really grabbed him. He told me he'd never seen a counselor or therapist, had never taken psychiatric medications, and wasn't about to start doing so now.

In fact, after his small reservoir of patience wore off, he sternly informed me that psychiatry was a "bullshit" field and that he'd be fine without my help. I asked him how his wife was going to feel if he didn't continue to meet with me. He told me to stay out of his marriage and mind my own business (which of course was his right to express). I apologized for the perceived intrusion and told him if at some point in the future he wanted to return, the door was open.

He softened a bit, we shook hands, and I wished him well as he left. I worried about him afterward because his anger was much higher than what most patients demonstrate, his new bride was so distraught, and he likely was using more coke than he admitted. Despite my concern, I didn't think I'd see him again.

Several days later, I got a call from his wife, who was anxious and asking for guidance. Since she was not my patient, and he had specifically refused to give me permission to discuss him with her or anybody else for that matter, I told her in general terms how someone might proceed with a relative who didn't want treatment. In her desperation, she called me again several days later, saying nothing had changed. After that call, I didn't hear from her again.

I thought about Ernesto over the next few months; although I've been called plenty of names, something was different about the intensity of his anger that was hard to shake, and I felt bad for his new wife.

A full two months had passed when, seemingly out of the blue, he called me. He immediately apologized for his rudeness during our meeting, then told me that he was broken and in need of help. When I saw him a couple of days later, his demeanor was completely different from our first meeting.

He said he realized that his wife was right—that his behavior had deteriorated significantly over the previous year and that cocaine played a role. He told me he was using more than he had initially reported. And although he'd thought it was helping him cope with the stress of work, he realized that cocaine was contributing to a downward spiral in his life and driving a wedge between him and his wife. He knew he'd acted terribly toward her and that she deserved better.

Plenty of patients have told me that they need to turn their lives around, and I'm often dubious about their actual ability to make significant changes despite their conviction in the moment. But something seemed different with Ernesto. He genuinely appeared to recognize the danger that lay ahead if he didn't change course, and he noted the pain he'd already caused his wife, who he repeatedly said was a wonderful woman. He told her that he'd take a drug test any time she wanted so she could feel secure about his sobriety.

As he came back for repeated visits, he opened up and shared more about his life. Ernesto had grown up in a working-class Irish American family in Boston. He played baseball and basketball on his high school teams and lived and breathed Boston and its sports teams. After making good—but not great—grades in high school, he went off to college without any clear career goals in mind. In college, he found a real passion for architecture and decided to go to graduate school in that field. It was only in grad school that he began using cocaine, and the first time he used it he knew he'd stumbled upon something that held immense appeal for him. He was too nervous about breaking the law to buy cocaine, so he would only use the drug when it surfaced at parties.

That changed after he began working in the architecture firm. Six months after taking the job, one of his co-workers told Ernesto that he had a safe, secure source of coke. That's all it took for Ernesto to begin using several times a week. And with that came the behavioral changes that his wife had noticed.

Once Ernesto and I began working together, he didn't just stop using cocaine: he remade himself into a better, healthier version of his previous self. Although he didn't care for AA, he launched into one of its Twelve Steps, trying to make amends to those he'd hurt through his cocaine use—especially his wife. He entirely stopped hanging around the several friends he had used cocaine with. He told his co-worker that he didn't want any more. After that, their interaction shifted to just a cordial working relationship. He worked hard to eliminate as much stress in his life as possible, although getting rid of all stress is impossible, especially for someone in an inherently stressful occupation.

As Ernesto made these changes, he became a nicer person. Eventually, he became genuinely transformed.

How Long Will I Need to Be Concerned about Drugs?

Perhaps the single question I am asked the most when someone considers giving up drugs is "Do I have to abstain from drugs for the rest of my life?" The usual teaching in medicine, psychiatry, and AA and NA states that "once an addict, always an addict," which means that—at least for people with full-blown addiction—the need for vigilance regarding drugs is lifelong and abstinence is the best course.

At the risk of invoking the ire of many people, although this teaching is common and it's certainly the safest way for anyone who's addicted or almost addicted to go through life, it is simply not always true that once someone has had a drug problem, that person can never return to safe, nonaddicted drug use. I see a seventy-five-year-old gentleman, for example, who for seven years was a homeless alcoholic (and kept some alcohol in him around the clock). He was eventually coaxed indoors by his primary care doctor and his girlfriend, and he sobered up. I came to know him roughly a decade after his homeless days, and by this point he would often have a glass of wine—sometimes two—with dinner and never got into trouble with alcohol again. I know of other similar stories, as well.

Some would say that this individual wasn't really an alcoholic but instead was a chronic abuser, because a real alcoholic (or addict) wouldn't be able to use again without returning to full-blown addiction. A lot of recent research supports this by showing that the neurochemistry of the brains of true alcoholics and addicts appears to be different, especially in the intensity of how they experience craving after they drink or use, which won't allow them to ever drink or use normally.

Much more important, people who are almost addicted are

different from those who are truly addicted. Their use never rises to the level of physical dependence and, by definition, never completely tears apart a life or several lives. It might be the case that someone who is almost addicted needs to remain completely drug free for life, but the fact is that experts don't really know.

I think the most important goal for someone who is almost addicted to drugs is to *not reenter the territory of problem-causing drug use.*

For many people, this mandate will absolutely mean that they shouldn't resume any drug use whatsoever. For others, it will mean that perhaps they might be able to use certain intoxicating substances someday, but that they should never again touch the drug that previously gave them problems. (As was the case for Alexa from chapter 3, who very rarely would use certain drugs, but knew that cocaine was too appealing and far too dangerous for her to ever risk using it again.)

I wish I could offer some completely black-and-white advice about using drugs that would be applicable for everyone, but doing so would probably be intellectually dishonest. You'll have to decide where to draw the line on what kind of presence that drugs—legal or not—can have in your life. You should remember, though, that drugs aren't like food—you *can* live without them. So if you have any doubt that they may be a problem for you, why wouldn't you stop using them? And if your drug of choice is illegal, breaking the law and risking arrest or the other dangers inherent in using street drugs are the best reasons to stop or to avoid starting again.

While you're learning how to live a healthy life without drugs, here are some steps that you can follow.

Don't Be Too Hard on Yourself over Slipups

Most people who are addicted to a substance and then stop using will slip up in their attempts to be drug free.

Even people who enter treatment programs are prone to relapse at some point, and many of them will go back into treatment. For example, one study that included people who had sought treatment for cocaine dependence up to five years earlier found that approximately 54 percent of them had used cocaine at some point afterward, and roughly 44 percent had returned to treatment.[102] This study, and many others I could cite, just confirms what I have witnessed in my years of working in addictions: namely, that addiction is a relapsing and remitting disease. I have seen people who have been in recovery from addiction for five, ten, or even fifteen years who then relapse, sometimes in the face of obvious stressors and sometimes for more mysterious reasons.

For someone who is almost addicted, whose relationship to drugs was never as unhealthy and damaging as it was for a person who was truly addicted, the principle is nonetheless the same. Even if you are successful in giving up your almost addiction, if you do slip up and use drugs at some point—whether or not you get into trouble in some way—don't beat yourself up over it. I certainly don't advocate merely shrugging off the use and acting like it's nothing, but on the other hand, I don't want to see people berating themselves when what happened is simply an expected event along the path to sobriety.

Take the time and energy that you could spend being angry or ashamed with your behavior and instead devote it to understanding what led to the slipup. Figure out what triggered the drug use and how you can keep it from happening again.

Maybe you need to find a healthy way to deal with a new stressor in your life. Perhaps you need to attend a few AA or NA meetings or to visit a mental health care provider again.

Stay Away from Places Where Drugs Are Being Used

This advice, which was discussed a few chapters ago, bears repeating. A crucial component in staying free of drugs is to simply stay away from them—and the people who are using them.

Does avoiding these high-risk situations mean you can't live your life absolutely any way that you choose? I'm sorry to say that the answer is probably yes. Living a drug-free life, given the role that drugs played in your life previously, requires you to consciously make changes that would seem strange to the almost addicted person who has not committed to change.

This means you can't keep going everywhere you could go when you were using drugs. You can't hang out with the same people. You'll have to get used to saying no on occasions when you would previously say yes. You may have to start potentially awkward conversations, like Ernesto did when he told his co-worker that he'd no longer be his customer.

Avoid Switching to Other Unhealthy Practices

I have seen plenty of patients who've given up one bad habit only to pick up another. For example, one person I've worked with has had free-floating addictive and self-abusive behaviors. She'd be smoking marijuana heavily, then give that up and become bulimic, then stop that and begin cutting herself, and then switch to alcohol. This kind of routine supports the notion of an "addictive personality," in which the person shifts from one addictive substance or behavior to another.

The literature offers some support for this concept of addiction. Howard Shaffer and colleagues have asserted that addiction is really a *syndromal* disorder.[103] What this means is that it is too simplistic to think of addiction as a behavior directed at only one substance of abuse. Instead, addiction is more of a syndrome, and when someone is vulnerable to becoming addicted, the addiction can be expressed in many ways or behaviors, with a common underlying explanation.

This would all apply to those who are almost addicted, too. If true, this picture of addiction explains why it is not uncommon for someone to kick one bad habit only to turn to another. When people beat a drug problem and live a healthy life in recovery, they will not—to use Shaffer's language—turn from one expression of addiction to another.

Whether or not Shaffer's hypothesis is correct—and I'm inclined to think it is—being healthy and living a full, complete life is the best way to ensure that stopping your drug use doesn't merely send you to the next bad habit.

Stay Attuned to Your Emotional Life

Many studies have concluded that negative emotions play a role in drug relapse after a period of sobriety.[104] That means you'll need to remain aware of how you're feeling, and whenever your emotions are in the gutter—and they eventually will be no matter how terrific your life is at other points—be aware that this might trigger thoughts of using.

If you don't remain tuned in to your emotions, uncomfortable feelings can easily blindside you. It's when you're not quite aware that you're feeling stressed or down that you might inadvertently turn to drugs to help you cope. But if you're always aware of how you feel, you are far more likely to be able to reach out for help in a healthy manner.

Prior to stopping cocaine, Ernesto was not particularly aware of his emotional state. Once he committed to sobriety, however, he definitely stayed keyed in to how he was feeling emotionally from day to day.

Don't Glamorize Your Past Drug Use

When looking back on past romantic relationships, many people focus only on the good times. They remember the wonderful gaze, the tender moments, the terrific sex, and the brilliance of mind, as opposed to all the cutting remarks, the failure to show up on time, or the repeated cheating.

Often, it's not too different with people who quit using drugs. I have known many people who formerly used drugs who had to constantly remind themselves that their good memories of the warm feelings paled in comparison to the pain and suffering their drug use caused, like the crimes they committed, the people they hurt, and the family members whose trust and love they abused.

Remember: if your drug use hadn't caused pain and suffering, you wouldn't have needed to quit using. So any time you begin to think fondly about "the good old days," immediately shift your thoughts to the pain, suffering, and fear that the drugs caused you and those around you.

Discuss Your Urges to Use

According to the tradition of the Sioux Native Americans, if someone had a vision that conferred the power to become a shaman (medicine man), telling others about the vision in any detail would cause the power it provided to disappear.

The same is true for everyone: narrating events saps them of their power and authority over people because they, and anyone who hears their story, gain some mastery and control over those events. The converse is that when things go unspoken, they retain their power.

If you start to think that you might want to go back to the drug that was at the center of your almost addiction, talk to those around you about it. Merely saying it out loud will almost magically take away some of the power that the substance holds over you. In addition, if you tell others about your urges to use, they'll no doubt relay the many reasons why you shouldn't risk using again, and this will even further reduce your chances of returning to the drug.

Be Careful Trying to Go It Alone

I've found that often when someone I've worked with begins to miss appointments or pulls back from engaging in conversation, drugs are involved. Given people's inherently social natures, being around other people often signifies health, whereas pulling back points toward the opposite.

Therefore, if you find yourself becoming isolated and avoiding others, seriously question whether you might be headed toward using drugs again. This is definitely a warning sign for many folks.

Stopping therapy or prescribed medications, or deciding that you know better than everyone around you about how to proceed is in all likelihood an unwise choice. It's also a potential warning sign that you are about to make other bad decisions such as returning to problematic drug use.

Watch Out When Major Life Changes Occur

If major events are approaching—even joyous ones like a wedding, the birth of a child, or holidays—beware that the inherent stress around any such events could trigger you to use. Other major changes that can cause significant stress include a death in the family, financial problems, or a new job.

Around these times, make doubly sure that you are employing the healthy coping skills that can keep you from turning to drugs for comfort.

Ernesto's Outcome

Ernesto very much loved his wife and enjoyed his job, and he didn't want his cocaine use to jeopardize either. He felt that turning away from the drug gave him a second chance at a good life.

After he stopped using, his demeanor changed for the better and he stayed drug-free. His wife stopped asking him to take drug tests after about six months. Around this time, another premier architecture firm in town that had admired his work offered him a job with better pay and even more responsibility. Seeing it as a chance to make a fresh start, Ernesto jumped at the opportunity.

He continued to stay free of drugs despite the stress of the job change and the new workload. After we worked together for about a year and a half, we both independently concluded that he had accomplished what he could in therapy, and we no longer needed to continue our visits. Somewhere Ernesto is out there designing buildings that are changing the city's skyline, and I hope his own horizon remains free of the drug that had threatened his happiness.

Final Thoughts

I have often told my students that if they want to write a best seller, they should start their book with a sentence that states either "Life is difficult" or "Life is painful." (It certainly worked well for M. Scott Peck in *The Road Less Traveled*.) I'm obviously not following my own advice, since I'm ending my book with this thought rather than opening with it.

Although I'm being a bit lighthearted with my students, my basic point is anything but. Even when life is going remarkably well, almost everyone experiences pain and sadness. And if you make the obvious explicit and state that life is painful, whoever you are with—or whoever is reading your book—is going to know that you're not just another person who is going to gloss over the hardship and try to BS your way through life. Instead, you introduce yourself as someone who is willing to stare at matters as they are and face situations head-on, without falsehood or pretense. You are someone who is ready and willing to roll up your sleeves and deal with life, however it presents itself.

What does this have to do with drug use? And why am I heading here now? I'm doing so because using drugs as a means of escape from a painful life has obvious appeal for many, many folks. But you already know that doing so can come at a price, perhaps a heavy one. You've taken this path before, and it didn't work. It's better to stick to another path in the future, one that involves other, healthier methods of dealing with the pain of life. Despite its many benefits, going drug free won't make your life easy or perfect. You're still going to face challenges. Your days will be difficult at times. That's because *life* is difficult. And life is painful. But you have other tools at your fingertips now that will get you through it.

Staying free of drugs need not feel like a burden, provided you have created a healthier, more enriching life for yourself. Being clean and able to face the world with honesty and openness can bring joyous gifts. Although doing so might feel daunting at first, taking this approach can (and should) be an invigorating and life-changing experience.

■ ◆ ■

notes

Introduction: Almost Addicted: The Basics

1. Office of National Drug Control Policy, "2009 National Survey on Drug Use and Health Highlights," 2010. www.whitehousedrugpolicy.gov /publications/html/nsduh.html.

2. Ibid.

3. University of Michigan Institute of Social Research, "Monitoring the Future—National Results on Adolescent Drug Use," 2011. http:// monitoringthefuture.org/pubs/monographs/mtf-overview2010.pdf.

4. National Institute on Drug Abuse, "Prescription Medications." www.nida.nih. gov/drugpages/prescription.html.

5. University of Michigan Institute of Social Research, "Monitoring the Future," 2011 [see n. 3].

6. NHS, "Statistics on Drug Misuse: England, 2010," 2011. www.ic.nhs.uk /webfiles/publications/003_Health_Lifestyles/Statistics_on_Drug _Misuse%20_England_2010.pdf.

7. European Monitoring Centre for Drugs and Drug Addiction, "Country Overview: Germany," 2010. www.emcdda.europa.eu/publications /country-overviews/de.

Chapter 1: *Almost* Addiction, but *Very Much* a Concern

8. R. Vandrey, A. Umbricht, and E. C. Strain, "Increased Blood Pressure Following Abrupt Cessation of Daily Cannabis Use," *Journal of Addiction Medicine* 5, no. 1 (2011): 16–20.

9. K. H. Levin, M. L. Copersino, S. J. Heishman, F. Liu, D. L. Kelly, D. L. Boggs, and D. A. Gorelick, "Cannabis Withdrawal Symptoms in Non-Treatment-Seeking Adult Cannabis Smokers," *Drug and Alcohol Dependence* 111, no. 1–2 (2010): 120–27.

10. Harvey A. Skinner, PhD, "Drug Use Questionnaire (DAST-20)," © 1982 by the Addiction Research Foundation. http://adai.washington.edu /instruments/pdf/Drug_Abuse_Screening_Test_105.pdf.

Chapter 2: Why Should I Change?

11. D. Henkel, "Unemployment and Substance Use: A Review of the Literature (1990–2010)," *Current Drug Abuse Reviews* 4, no. 1 (2011): 4–27.

12. D. J. Gascon and H. A. Spiller, "Relationship of Unemployment Rate and Rate of Opiate Exposure in Kentucky," *Journal of Psychoactive Drugs* 41, no. 1 (2009): 99–102.

13. Office of National Drug Control Policy, "Marijuana Facts and Figures." www.whitehousedrugpolicy.gov/drugfact/marijuana/marijuana _ff.html#arrests.

14. European Monitoring Centre for Drugs and Drug Addiction, "Drug Law Offences, 1995 to 2008." www.emcdda.europa.eu/stats10/dlotab1a.

15. Harvard University, "Drug/Alcohol and Smoking Policies." https:// intranet.seas.harvard.edu/human-resources/policies-and-procedures /drug-alcohol-policy.

16. R. N. Hansen, G. Oster, J. Edelsberg, G. E. Woody, and S. D. Sullivan, "Economic Costs of Nonmedical Use of Prescription Opioids," *Clinical Journal of Pain* 27, no. 3 (2011): 194–202.

17. Robert Wood Johnson Foundation, "Substance Abuse—The Nation's Number One Health Problem," 2001. www.rwjf.org/files/publications /other/SubstanceAbuseChartbook.pdf.

18. L. A. Benishek, K. C. Kirby, and K. L. Dugosh, "Prevalence and Frequency of Problems of Concerned Family Members with a Substance-Using Loved One," *American Journal of Drug and Alcohol Abuse* 37, no. 2 (2011): 82–88.

19. A. J. Heinz, J. Wu, K. Witkiewitz, D. H. Epstein, and K. L. Preston, "Marriage and Relationship Closeness as Predictors of Cocaine and Heroin Use," *Addictive Behaviors* 34, no. 3 (2009): 258–63.

20. Drug Abuse Warning Network, "Highlights of the 2009 Drug Abuse Warning Network (DAWN) Findings on Drug-Related Emergency Department Visits," 2010. http://oas.samhsa.gov/2k10/DAWN034 /EDHighlights.htm.

21. Drug Abuse Warning Network, "Drug-Related Emergency Department Visits Involving Pharmaceutical Misuse and Abuse by Older Adults," 2010. http://oas.samhsa.gov/2k10/dawn018/Pharma50plus.htm.

22. Center for Behavioral Health Statistics and Quality, "State Estimates of Drunk and Drugged Driving," National Survey on Drug Use and Health, 2010. http://oas.samhsa.gov/2k10/205/DruggedDriving.htm.

23. L. Arseneault, M. Cannon, R. Poulton, R. Murray, A. Caspi, and T. E. Moffitt, "Cannabis Use in Adolescence and Risk for Adult Psychosis: Longitudinal Prospective Study, *British Medical Journal* 325, no. 7374 (2002), 1212–13.

24. S. Zammit, P. Allebeck, S. Andreasson, I. Lundberg, and G. Lewis, "Self Reported Cannabis Use as a Risk Factor for Schizophrenia in Swedish Conscripts of 1969: Historical Cohort Study." *British Medical Journal* 325, no. 7374 (2002), 1199.

25. P. Y. Le Bec, M. Fatséas, C. Denis, E. Lavie, and M. Auriacombe, "Cannabis and Psychosis: Search of a Causal Link through a Critical and Systematic Review," *Encephale* 35, no. 4 (2009), 377–85.

26. G. C. Patton, C. Coffey, J. B. Carlin, L. Degenhardt, M. Lynskey, and W. Hall, "Cannabis Use and Mental Health in Young People: Cohort Study, *British Medical Journal* 325, no. 7374 (2002): 1195–98.

27. Center for Behavioral Health Statistics and Quality, "Illicit Drug Use among Persons Arrested for Serious Crimes," National Survey on Drug Use and Health, 2005. http://oas.samhsa.gov/2k5/arrests/arrests.htm.

28. Office of National Drug Control Policy, "Fact Sheet—2008 ADAM Report," 2009. http://whitehousedrugpolicy.gov/pdf/ADAMII_Fact_sheet_2008.pdf.

Chapter 3: When the Past Influences the Present

29. M. J. Kreek, D. A. Nielsen, E. R., Butelman, and K. S. LaForge, "Genetic Influences on Impulsivity, Risk Taking, Stress Responsivity and Vulnerability to Drug Abuse and Addiction," *Nature Neuroscience* 8, no. 11 (2005): 1450–57.

30. Ibid.

31. J. L. Richardson, B. Radziszewska, C. W. Dent, and B. R. Flay, "Relationship between After-School Care of Adolescents and Substance Use, Risk Taking, Depressed Mood, and Academic Achievement," *Pediatrics* 92, no. 1 (1993): 32–38.

32. G. Gerra, C. Leonardi, E. Cortese, A. Zaimovic, G. Dell'agnello, M. Manfredini, L. Somaini, F. Petracca, V. Caretti, M. A. Raggi, and C. Donnini, "Childhood Neglect and Parental Care Perception in Cocaine Addicts: Relation with Psychiatric Symptoms and Biological Correlates," *Neuroscience and Biobehavioral Reviews* 33, no. 4 (2009): 601–10.

33. J. M. Hussey, J. J. Chang, and J. B. Kotch, "Child Maltreatment in the United States: Prevalence, Risk Factors, and Adolescent Health Consequences," *Pediatrics* 118, no. 3 (2006): 933–42.

34. R. A. Harvey and P. C. Champe, eds., *Lippincott's Illustrated Reviews, Pharmacology, 4th* ed. (Baltimore: Lippincott Williams & Wilkins, 2008).

35. F. E. Atianjoh, B. Ladenheim, I. N. Krasnova, and J. L. Cadet, "Amphetamine Causes Dopamine Depletion and Cell Death in the Mouse Olfactory Bulb," *European Journal of Pharmacology* 589, no. 1–3 (2008): 94–97.

Chapter 4: Double Trouble: Almost Addiction and Mental Health Issues

36. US Department of Health and Human Services, "Results from the 2009 National Survey on Drug Use and Health: Mental Health Findings," 2010. www.oas.samhsa.gov/NSDUH/2k9NSDUH/MH/2K9MHResults. pdf.

37. Hazelden Foundation, "Frequently Asked Questions About Co-Occurring Disorders," Behavioral Health Evolution, www.bhevolution.org/public/overview_faqs.page.

38. National Institute on Drug Abuse, "Comorbidity: Addiction and Other Mental Illnesses," 2010. http://drugabuse.gov/PDF/RRComorbidity.pdf.

39. L. Davis, A. Uezato, J. M. Newell, and E. Frazier, "Major Depression and Comorbid Substance Use Disorders," *Current Opinion in Psychiatry* 21, no. 1 (2008): 14–18.

40. D. A. Regier, M. E. Farmer, D. S. Rae, B. Z. Locke, S. J. Keith, L. L. Judd, and F. K. Goodwin, "Comorbidity of Mental Disorders with Alcohol and Other Drug Abuse. Results from the Epidemiologic Catchment Area (ECA) Study," *Journal of the American Medical Association* 264, no. 19 (1990): 2511–18.

41. M. S. Swartz, H. R. Wagner, J. W. Swanson, T. S. Stroup, J. P. McEvoy, M. McGee, D. D. Miller, F. Reimherr, A. Khan, J. Cañive, and J. Lieberman, "Substance Use and Psychosocial Functioning in Schizophrenia among New Enrollees in the NIMH CATIE Study," *Psychiatric Services* 57 (2006): 1110–16.

42. K. R. Merikangas, H. S. Akiskal, J. Angst, P. E. Greenberg, R. M. Hirschfeld, M. Petukhova, and R. C. Kessler, "Lifetime and 12-Month Prevalence of Bipolar Spectrum Disorder in the National Comorbidity Survey Replication," *Archives of General Psychiatry* 64, no. 5 (2007): 543–52; D. A. Regier, "Comorbidity of Mental Disorders with Alcohol and Other Drug Abuse," [see chap. 4, n. 40].

43. R. M. Bray, M. R. Pemberton, M. E. Lane, L. L. Hourani, M. J. Mattiko, and L. A. Babeu, "Substance Use and Mental Health Trends among U.S. Military Active Duty Personnel: Key Findings from the 2008 DoD Health Behavior Survey," *Military Medicine* 175, no.6 (2010): 390–99.

44. T. E. Wilens, M. Martelon, G. Joshi, C. Bateman, R. Fried, C. Petty, and J. Biederman, "Does ADHD Predict Substance-Use Disorders? A 10-Year Follow-Up Study of Young Adults with ADHD," *Journal of the American Academy of Child and Adolescent Psychiatry* 50, no. 6 (2011): 545–53.

45. I. L. Petrakis, R. Rosenheck, and R. Desai, "Substance Use Comorbidity among Veterans with Posttraumatic Stress Disorder and Other Psychiatric Illness," *American Journal on Addictions* 20, no. 3 (2011): 185–89.

46. T. E. Wilens, J. Biederman, A. M. Abrantes, and T. J. Spencer, "Clinical Characteristics of Psychiatrically Referred Adolescent Outpatients with Substance Use Disorder," *Journal of the American Academy of Child and Adolescent Psychiatry* 36, no. 7 (1997): 941–47.

47. R. Modrzejewska, "Comorbidity in Adolescence: Simultaneous Declaration of Depressive, Eating, Obsessive-Compulsive Symptoms and Use of Psychoactive Substances in the General Population of 17 Year Old Students in a Big City," *Psychiatria Polska* 44, no. 5 (2010): 651–63.

48. R. J. Stowell and T. W. Estroff, "Psychiatric Disorders in Substance-Abusing Adolescent Inpatients," *Journal of the American Academy of Child and Adolescent Psychiatry* 31, no. 6 (1992): 1036–40.

49. Zammit et al., "Self-Reported Cannabis Use as a Risk Factor for Schizophrenia," [see chap. 2, n. 24].

50. Centers for Disease Control and Prevention, "Attention-Deficit/Hyperactivity Disorder (ADHD): Data and Statistics," 2010. www.cdc.gov/ncbddd/adhd/data.html.

51. R. A. Barkley, M. Fischer, L. Smallish, and K. Fletcher, "Does the Treatment of Attention-Deficit/Hyperactivity Disorder with Stimulants Contribute to Drug Use/Abuse? A 13-Year Prospective Study, *Pediatrics* 111, no. 1 (2003): 97–109.

52. T. E. Wilens, J. Adamson, M. C. Monuteaux, S. V. Faraone, M. Schillinger, D. Westerberg, and J. Biederman, "Effect of Prior Stimulant Treatment for Attention-Deficit/Hyperactivity Disorder on Subsequent Risk for Cigarette Smoking and Alcohol and Drug Use Disorders in Adolescents," *Archives of Pediatrics & Adolescent Medicine* 162, no. 10 (2008): 916–21.

53. S. Dennison, "Substance Use Disorders in Individuals with Co-Occuring Psychiatric Disorders," in *Substance Abuse: A Comprehensive Textbook*, 5th ed., edited by P. Ruiz and E. Strain (Baltimore: Lippincott Williams & Wilkins, 2011).

54. M. Bruce, N. Scott, P. Shine, and M. Lader, "Anxiogenic Effect of Caffeine in Patients with Anxiety Disorders," *Archives of General Psychiatry* 49, no. 11 (1992): 867–69.

55. S. A. Saeed, D. J. Antonacci, and R. M. Bloch, "Exercise, Yoga, and Meditation for Depressive and Anxiety Disorders," *American Family Physician* 81, no. 8 (2010): 981–86.

56. F. S. Radhakishun, J. M. van Ree, and B. H. Westerink, "Scheduled Eating Increases Dopamine Release in the Nucleus Accumbens of Food-Deprived Rats as Assessed with On-Line Brain Dialysis," *Neuroscience Letters* 85, no. 3 (1988): 351–56; L. Hernandez and B. G. Hoebel, "Food Reward and Cocaine Increase Extracellular Dopamine in the Nucleus Accumbens as Measured by Microdialysis," *Life Sciences* 42, no. 18 (1988): 1705–12; D. Sutoo and K. Akiyama, "The Mechanism by Which Exercise Modifies Brain Function," *Physiology & Behavior* 60, no. 1 (1996): 177–81.

Chapter 5: Recognizing an Invisible Problem

57. D. Brooke, G. Edwards, and C. Taylor, "Addiction as an Occupational Hazard: 144 Doctors with Drug and Alcohol Problems," *British Journal of Addiction* 86, no. 8 (1991): 1011–16.

58. S. Van Hook, S. K. Harris, T. Brooks, P. Carey, R. Kossack, J. Kulig, and J. R. Knight, "The 'SIX T's': Barriers to Screening Teens for Substance Abuse in Primary Care," *Journal of Adolescent Health* 40, no. 5 (2007): 456–61.

59. P. D. Friedmann, D. McCullough, and R. Saitz, "Screening and Intervention for Illicit Drug Abuse: A National Survey of Primary Care Physicians and Psychiatrists," *Archives of Internal Medicine* 161, no. 2 (2001): 248–51.

60. K. S. Yarnall, K. I. Pollak, T. Ostbye, K. M. Krause, and J. L. Michener, "Primary Care: Is There Enough Time for Prevention?" *American Journal of Public Health* 93, no. 4 (2003): 635–41.

61. P. Nilsen, E. Kaner and T. F. Babor, "Brief Intervention, Three Decades On," *Nordic Studies on Alcohol and Drugs* 25 (2008): 453–67.

Chapter 6: Confronting and Solving a Loved One's Almost Addiction

62. Adapted from Al-Anon Family Groups, "How do you know if you are affected by someone's drinking?" www.al-anon.alateen.org/affected-by-someones-drinking.

Chapter 7: Unsafe at Any Age: Almost Addicted Across the Life Span

63. R. C. Kessler, P. Berglund, O. Demler, R. Jin, K. R. Merikangas, E. E. Walters, "Lifetime Prevalence and Age-of-Onset Distributions of DSM-IV Disorders in the National Comorbidity Survey Replication," *Archives of General Psychiatry* 62, no. 6 (2005): 593–602.

64. University of Michigan Institute of Social Research, "Monitoring the Future," [see chap. 1, n. 3].

65. R. W. Hingson, T. Heeren, and M. R. Winter, "Age at Drinking Onset and Alcohol Dependence: Age at Onset, Duration, and Severity," *Archives of Pediatrics & Adolescent Medicine* 160, no. 7 (2006): 739–46; Substance Abuse and Mental Health Services Administration, "Results from the 2009 National Survey on Drug Use and Health: Volume I. Summary of National Findings," 2010. http://oas.samhsa.gov/nsduh/2k9nsduh/2k9resultsp.pdf.

66. M. G. Bossong and R. J. Niesink, "Adolescent Brain Maturation, the Endogenous Cannabinoid System and the Neurobiology of Cannabis-Induced Schizophrenia," *Progress in Neurobiology* 92, no. 3 (2010): 370–85.

67. B. J. Casey, S. Getz, and A. Galvan, "The Adolescent Brain," *Developmental Review* 28, no. 1 (2008): 62–77.

68. N. L. Schramm-Sapyta, Q. D. Walker, J. M. Caster, E. D. Levin, and C. M. Kuhn, "Are Adolescents More Vulnerable to Drug Addiction Than Adults? Evidence from Animal Models," *Psychopharmacology* 206, no. 1 (2009): 1–21.

69. B. D. Peters, J. Blaas, and L. de Haan, "Diffusion Tensor Imaging in the Early Phase of Schizophrenia: What Have We Learned?" *Journal of Psychiatric Research* 44, no. 15 (2010): 993–1004.

70. T. Rubino, E. Zamberletti, and D. Parolaro, "Adolescent Exposure to Cannabis as a Risk Factor for Psychiatric Disorders," *Journal of Psychopharmacology* 26, no. 1, (2011): 177–88.

71. Centers for Disease Control and Prevention, "Attention-Deficit/ Hyperactivity Disorder" 2010. [see chap. 4, n. 50].

72. G. Polanczyk, M. S. de Lima, B. L. Horta, J. Biederman, and L. A. Rohde, "The Worldwide Prevalence of ADHD: A Systematic Review and Metaregression Analysis," *American Journal of Psychiatry* 164 (2007): 942–48.

73. P. Miller and M. Plant, "Parental Guidance about Drinking: Relationship with Teenage Psychoactive Substance Use," *Journal of Adolescence* 33, no. 1 (2010): 55–68.

74. National Center on Addiction and Substance Abuse at Columbia University, "The Importance of Family Dinners IV," 2007. www.casacolumbia.org, downloadable file 30dqhuyg.pdf.

75. Substance Abuse and Mental Health Services Administration, "An Examination of Trends in Illicit Drug Use among Adults Aged 50 to 59 in the United States," 2009. http://oas.samhsa.gov/2k9/OlderAdults /OAS_data_review_OlderAdults.pdf.

76. Substance Abuse and Mental Health Services Administration, "Results from the 2008 National Survey on Drug Use and Health: National Findings," 2009. http://oas.samhsa.gov/nsduh/2k8nsduh/2k8Results .cfm#2.4

77. D. W. Kaufman, J. P. Kelly, L. Rosenberg, T. E. Anderson, and A. A. Mitchell, "Recent Patterns of Medication Use in the Ambulatory Adult Population of the United States: The Slone Survey," *Journal of the American Medical Association* 287, no. 3 (2002): 337–44.

78. T. Jorgensen, S. Johansson, A. Kennerfalk, M. A. Wallander, and K. Svardsudd, "Prescription Drug Use, Diagnoses, and Healthcare Utilization among the Elderly," *Annals of Pharmacotherapy* 35, no. 9 (2001): 1004–9.

Chapter 8: Time for a Change: Helping Yourself

79. J. R. Cornelius, D. B. Clark, M. Reynolds, L. Kirisci, and R. Tarter, "Early Age of First Sexual Intercourse and Affiliation with Deviant Peers Predict Development of SUD: A Prospective Longitudinal Study," *Addictive Behaviors* 32, no. 4 (2007): 850–54.

80. T. Korhonen, A. C. Huizink, D. M. Dick, L. Pulkkinen, R. J. Rose,. and J. Kaprio, "Role of Individual, Peer and Family Factors in the Use of Cannabis and Other Illicit Drugs: A Longitudinal Analysis among Finnish Adolescent Twins," *Drug and Alcohol Dependence* 97, no. 1–2 (2008): 33–43.

81. G. G. Homish, K. E. Leonard, and J. R. Cornelius, "Individual, Partner and Relationship Factors Associated with Non-Medical Use of Prescription Drugs," *Addiction* 105, no. 8 (2010): 1457–65.

82. C. B. Taylor, J. F. Sallis, and R. Needle, "The Relation of Physical Activity and Exercise to Mental Health," *Public Health Reports* 100, no. 2 (1985): 195–202.

83. K. K. Roessler, "Exercise Treatment for Drug Abuse—A Danish Pilot Study," *Scandinavian Journal of Public Health* 38, no. 6 (2010): 664–69.

84. F. L. Vázquez, "Psychoactive Substance Use and Dependence among Spanish University Students: Prevalence, Correlates, Polyconsumption, and Comorbidity with Depression," *Psychological Reports* 106, no. 1 (2010): 297–313.

85. T. Wichstrøm and L. Wichstrøm, "Does Sports Participation during Adolescence Prevent Later Alcohol, Tobacco and Cannabis use?" *Addiction* 104, no. 1 (2009): 138–49; T. Korhonen, U. M. Kujala, R. J. Rose, and J. Kaprio, "Physical Activity in Adolescence as a Predictor of Alcohol and Illicit Drug Use in Early Adulthood: A Longitudinal Population-Based Twin Study," *Twin Research and Human Genetics* 12, no. 3 (2009): 261–68.

86. A. Sanchez-Villegas, M. Delgado-Rodriguez, A. Alonso, J. Schlatter, F. Lahortiga, L. Serra-Majem, and M. A. Martinez-Gonzalez, "Association of the Mediterranean Dietary Pattern with the Incidence of Depression," *Archive of General Psychiatry* 66, no. 10 (2009): 1090–98.

87. P. Henríquez Sánchez, C. Ruano, J. de Irala, M. Ruiz-Canela, M. A. Martínez-González, and A. Sánchez-Villegas, "Adherence to the Mediterranean Diet and Quality of Life in the SUN Project," *European Journal of Clinical Nutrition* 66, no. 3 (2012): 360–68.

88. L. McMillan, L. Owen, M. Kras, .A. Scholey, "Behavioural Effects of a 10-Day Mediterranean Diet. Results from a Pilot Study Evaluating Mood and Cognitive Performance," *Appetite* 56, no. 1 (2011): 143–47.

89. S. P. Barrett, C. Darredeau, and R. O. Pihl, "Patterns of Simultaneous Polysubstance Use in Drug Using University Students," *Human Psychopharmacology* 21, no. 4 (2006): 255–63.

90. L. H. Powell, L. Shahabi, and C. E. Thoresen, "Religion and Spirituality. Linkages to Physical Health," *American Psychologist* 58, no. 1 (2003): 36–52.

91. A. Heinz, D. H. Epstein, K. L. Preston, "Spiritual/Religious Experiences and In-Treatment Outcome in an Inner-City Program for Heroin and Cocaine Dependence," *Journal of Psychoactive Drugs* 39, no. 1 (2007): 41–49.

92. J. R. Cornelius, et al., "Early Age of First Sexual Intercourse and Affiliation with Deviant Peers Predict Development of SUD [see chap. 8, n. 79].

Chapter 9: Time for a Change: Getting Help from Others

93. A. Baker, N. K. Lee, M. Claire, T. J. Lewin, T. Grant, S. Pohlman, J. B. Saunders, and F. Kay-Lambkin, "Brief Cognitive Behavioural Interventions for Regular Amphetamine Users: A Step in the Right Direction," *Addiction* 100, no. 3 (2005): 367–78.

94. J. Bernstein, E. Bernstein, K. Tassiopoulos, T. Heeren, S. Levenson, and R. Hingson, "Brief Motivational Intervention at a Clinic Visit Reduces Cocaine and Heroin Use," *Drug and Alcohol Dependence* 77, no. 1 (2005): 49–59.

95. C. Breslin, S. Li, K. Sdao-Jarvie, E. Tupker, and V. Ittig-Deland, "Brief Treatment for Young Substance Abusers: A Pilot Study in an Addiction Treatment Setting," *Psychology of Addictive Behaviors* 16, no. 1 (2002): 10–16.

96. K. T. Mueser, R. E. Drake, W. Turner, and M. S. McGovern, "Comorbid Substance Use Disorders and Psychiatric Disorders," in *Substance Abuse: What the Science Shows, and What We Should Do About It*, edited by W. R. Miller and K. M. Carroll (New York: Guilford Press, 2006).

97. W. R. Miller and S. Rollnick, *Motivational Interviewing: Preparing People for Change* (New York: Guilford Press, 2002).

98. E. Evans, D. Huang, and Y. I. Hser, "High-Risk Offenders Participating in Court-Supervised Substance Abuse Treatment: Characteristics, Treatment Received, and Factors Associated with Recidivism," *Journal of Behavioral Health Services & Research* 38, no. 4 (2011): 510–25.

99. A. Kaskutas, J. Bond, and K. Humphreys, "Social Networks as Mediators of the Effect of Alcoholics Anonymous," *Addiction* 97, no. 7 (2002): 891–900.

100. Heinz, Epstein, and Preston, "Spiritual/Religious Experiences and In-Treatment Outcome," [see chap. 8, n. 91].

Chapter 10: After Almost Addiction—Now What? Living without Drugs

101. A. T. McLellan, J. R. McKay, R. Forman, J. Cacciola, and J. Kemp, "Reconsidering the Evaluation of Addiction Treatment: From Retrospective Follow-Up to Concurrent Recovery Monitoring," *Addiction* 100, no. 4 (2005): 447–58.

102. C. E. Grella, Y. I. Hser, and S. C. Hsieh, "Predictors of Drug Treatment Re-Entry Following Relapse to Cocaine Use in DATOS," *Journal of Substance Abuse Treatment* 25, no. 3 (2003): 145–54.

103. H. J. Shaffer, D. A. LaPlante, R. A. LaBrie, R. C. Kidman, A. N. Donato, and M. V. Stanton, "Toward a Syndrome Model of Addiction: Multiple Expressions, Common Etiology," *Harvard Review of Psychiatry* 12 (2004): 367–74.

104. J. R. McKay, "Studies of Factors in Relapse to Alcohol, Drug and Nicotine Use: A Critical Review of Methodologies and Findings," *Journal of Studies on Alcohol and Drugs* 60, no. 4 (1999): 566–76.

about the authors

J. Wesley "Wes" Boyd, MD, PhD, is on the faculty in Psychiatry at Harvard Medical School, is a staff psychiatrist at Children's Hospital Boston and at Cambridge Health Alliance (CHA), and is the founder and co-director of the Human Rights and Asylum Clinic at CHA. At Children's Hospital Boston he works in the Adolescent Substance Abuse Program. At Cambridge, he is a psychiatrist for one of the principal training and teaching teams whose focus is on the interface between substance use disorders and general adult psychiatry.

Dr. Boyd graduated cum laude with a BA from Yale in philosophy. He then attended the University of North Carolina at Chapel Hill where he received an MA in philosophy, a PhD in religion and culture, and a medical degree. Following graduate school and medical school, he completed a residency in psychiatry at Cambridge Hospital/Harvard Medical School and also completed a Fellowship in Medical Ethics through the Department of Social Medicine (now called the Department of Global Health and Social Medicine) at Harvard Medical School.

He has taught medical ethics and the humanities in various venues and currently teaches medical ethics to medical students and psychiatry residents at Harvard. He also teaches a popular freshman seminar at Harvard College titled "Psychology of Religion." He writes for both lay and academic audiences on issues of health care justice as well as humanistic aspects of medicine. His writing has appeared in the *Journal of the American Medical Association, New England Journal of Medicine,* the *Boston Globe,* and The Huffington Post, among other media outlets. His work has been reported by *Time*, the *Wall Street Journal*, CBS, CNN, and other major media outlets.

Eric Metcalf, MPH, is a consumer health writer and educator based in Indianapolis, Indiana. He has coauthored or contributed to dozens of books on health and fitness and has written extensively for online outlets, including WebMD, and magazines. He's also produced a number of medical-themed essays and stories for public radio.

▪ ◆ ▪